SUGAR BUSTERS!™

SUGAR BUSTERS!™

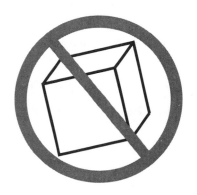

CUT SUGAR TO TRIM FAT

H. LEIGHTON STEWARD

MORRISON C. BETHEA, M.D.

SAMUEL S. ANDREWS, M.D.

LUIS A. BALART, M.D.

BALLANTINE BOOKS · NEW YORK

A Ballantine Book
Published by The Ballantine Publishing Group

Updates and revisions copyright © 1998 by Sugar Busters, L.L.C.

http://www.randomhouse.com
http://www.sugarbusters.com

Library of Congress Cataloging-in-Publication Data
Sugar busters! / H. Leighton Steward . . . [et al.].
    p.   cm.
    Includes index.
    ISBN 0-345-42558-8 (alk. paper)
    1. Refined carbohydrates—Pathophysiology. 2. Insulin—Pathophysi-
ology. 3. Sugar-free diet. I. Steward, H. Leighton.
RC627.R43S84   1998   98-9669
613.2'83—dc21   CIP

Manufactured in the United States of America

First Edition: May 1998

22 23 24 25 26 27 28 29 30

Dedicated to our very enthusiastic and supportive wives, Lynda Steward, Brenda Bethea, Linda Andrews, and Muffin Balart (whole-grain, of course).

Contents

Foreword

SUGAR BUSTERS! has revolutionized the way New Orleans, Louisiana, eats!

Over the past several years I personally have witnessed local interest and enthusiasm for the SUGAR BUSTERS! lifestyle as it built to its present pounding crescendo. It is difficult to ignore a way of eating that monopolizes conversation at cocktail parties, has shelf space in every appropriate retail outlet, and dominates many restaurants' menus in the #1 food city in the world.

SUGAR BUSTERS! devotees are a diverse group. They are men and women, professional and working class, soccer moms and sorority girls. Some are seriously obese, and others need to lose a few extra pounds. But all followers of the SUGAR BUSTERS! lifestyle have one thing in common . . . the fierce desire to decrease overall body fat and improve their health through smart nutrition.

I use the word "lifestyle" as opposed to "diet" when referring to SUGAR BUSTERS! because "diet" sounds restrictive and intimidating, and SUGAR BUSTERS! is just the opposite. SUGAR BUSTERS! is the most flexible eating plan I've ever known, as it allows me to eat most foods in conventional portion sizes.

As a restaurateur, I consider this good news because I am professionally obligated to eat almost every meal, every day, in a New Orleans restaurant (yes, it *is* good work if you can get it!), but left unchecked, eating with such reckless abandon is asking for trouble. Herein lies the beauty of SUGAR BUSTERS! because most home and restaurant recipes can be easily adapted to meet the SUGAR BUSTERS! requirements. Lean meats, chicken and fish, fresh vegetables, fresh fruit, the right (low insulin-producing) carbohydrates, and even red wine are all within the parameters of the plan.

For many years I have watched restaurant guests become increasingly concerned about their health and eating habits. Salads are more popular, and grilled fish is our best-selling item. Yet dessert sales continue to grow! What's happening? Customers keep score. If they're dining out tonight, they'll eat a light lunch—perhaps a piece of fresh grilled fish or an entrée salad, or to save room for dessert, the guest might choose a lighter entrée.

That's what SUGAR BUSTERS! offers: the flexibility to make good choices from a wide selection of menu items without compromising variety, freshness, or flavor. And even the occasional dessert is okay. Remember, this is a low-sugar lifestyle, not a no-sugar lifestyle!

New Orleans is a food city, and cooking is our favorite sport! It is difficult to consistently ignore Sweet Potato Catfish at Red Fish Grill, Fennel Crusted Tuna at Bacco, or Barbecued Shrimp at Mr. B's Bistro. But within the parameters of the SUGAR BUSTERS! lifestyle, each of these signature New Orleans dishes and many others are well within the plan!

SUGAR BUSTERS! is the newest and best approach to transforming the way America eats. The plan is flexible and fun, and its renowned authors present their case in plain language supported by research dating back twenty years. Each of the authors practices what he preaches and has lived the SUGAR BUSTERS! lifestyle for a number of years. Best of all, SUGAR BUSTERS! really works!

So what are YOU waiting for? Eat, Drink, (red wine, of course), & Be Merry!

Ralph O. Brennan

Owner, Red Fish Grill, Bacco, Mr. B's Bistro

Past Chairman and President of the National Restaurant Association (1995–96)

New Orleans, Louisiana

Preface

Why another book on dieting or how to eat? Haven't they all been written? Nearly all overlook the profound effect of one of the body's most powerful hormones—*insulin*. This was the principal message in the original SUGAR BUSTERS!, which has now been proven effective by tens of thousands of followers who have so successfully lost weight, improved their blood chemistries, or, very importantly, have controlled their diabetes much better.

Because most diets are aimed at weight loss, they have historically recommended reducing calories and/or fat; this practice is unnatural to an affluent society or even the Eskimos of North America. America is in dire need of a way of eating (and drinking) that will allow its people to consume reasonable quantities of food that can improve their daily enjoyment of life. At the same time, this new way of eating should eliminate unwanted quantities of weight and, more importantly, the adverse effects current eating habits have on blood cholesterol, triglycerides, and causing, or negatively affecting, diabetes.

Is a diet really needed to enhance everybody's health and performance? A large percentage of our population is faced with the daily decisions and stress levels that were afforded only to some of the country's top leaders just a few decades ago. In our lives today, at home and work and in between, we are faced with constant demands: phone calls, faxes, computer problems and opportunities, high speed, close-quarter traffic situations, and dawn-to-dawn media bombardments of local and worldwide murders, pestilence, catastrophes, and wars. So, we all need to be ready to best handle the mental and physical demands each day presents.

Four authors? Gasp! How could it work? Well, we hope it did; you will have to be the judge. We thought it should because we are all excited and highly motivated to get a message out that should actually benefit mankind—and mankind certainly is in need of some help in the area of eating habits.

One author, a Fortune 500 CEO, is in his sixties and slim. He has been eating the way this book recommends for over five years and is still twenty pounds down from his starting weight and has significantly improved his blood chemistry. All this at an average of 3,100 calories a day!

Of our three doctor authors, we have a cardiovascular surgeon, an endocrinologist, and a gastroenterologist. These are not ordinary doctors. Our heart surgeon has been voted the number-one cardiovascular surgeon in the greater New Orleans area by his peers, the most respected vote a doctor can receive. The endocrinologist is a member of the Audubon Internal Medicine Group at the largest hospital in New Orleans. Our gastroenterologist, a member of the Center for Digestive Diseases at Tenet's Memorial Medical Center in New Orleans, is an expert in liver function and metabolism. He is extremely key in verifying the connections between various hormonal secretions and the liver, where cholesterol is manufactured.

Acknowledgments

The original introduction to the advantages of a painless, but beneficial, way of eating came to us through Victor Rice and his wife, Corinne. The inspiration for their way of eating came from Michel Montignac in *Dine Out & Lose Weight*. The negative effects of sugar had actually been described in 1976 by William Dufty in *Sugar Blues*. Interestingly enough, although Dufty recognized insulin as having bad effects on the body and mind, neither he nor Montignac sufficiently described why or how insulin wreaks such havoc on our bodies or the tremendous benefits to diabetics of eliminating certain carbohydrates from their diets. Yet, without their priming, what follows may have never begun.

I | Introduction

- If you enjoy eating, this is a good-news book.
- If you choose to eat out frequently or if your employment requires it, this is a good-news book.
- If you want your blood chemistry to improve while you continue to eat more savory foods, this is a good-news book.
- If you want to lose significant quantities of weight, this is a good-news book.
- If you are diabetic, this is a good-news book.
- All these benefits are possible while you are feeling and functioning better in the process.

We are going to propose a way of eating that will allow you to eat most foods in normal quantities, possibly even in larger quantities than you presently consume. You can have three full meals a day and even appropriate snacks. There will not be many things you cannot eat, but there will be certain combinations you should definitely avoid. What you need to avoid most will be foods or combinations of foods that require the secretion of large amounts of insulin to regulate your blood sugar. By simply doing this, you can get slimmer and healthier simultaneously.

We would like to write a thick, fine-print book about all this good news, but a book that covers the weight-loss implications of eating well has already been written by Michel Montignac (1986) of France, and William Dufty (1976) has described the evil effects of sugar itself in his *Sugar Blues*.

There are now other published books that also recommend a higher percentage of protein in one's diet, but they generally are so technical or all-inclusive that they end up confusing the reader. Nearly all miss one of the most important factors in successful, extended weight loss, which is the ability of certain carbohydrates to increase dramatically your body's need for insulin.

We believe, in today's hurried and complex world, that most readers actually prefer succinct and straightforward summaries of what works, what does not, and why, plus a few reliable charts and graphs that prove how and why it works. Chapter XVII answers our readers' most frequently asked questions. We also have provided a layman's glossary to assist you in understanding some of the technical terms often required to describe properly various processes or facts. In addition, so as not to keep you in curious suspense for a hundred pages or more, we want to give you the essence of our findings in this introduction.

Let's get to the point. *Sugar is toxic!* Sugar? Some sugar? Most sugar? All sugar? Toxic? Well, we will say that *refined* sugar in any significant quantity is toxic to many human bodies, and it certainly helps make many bodies fat. Moreover, significant quantities of sugar are derived in our digestive systems from carbohydrates and starches. Certain of these foods cause a definite strain on the health of the body, probably the mind, and certainly the waistline. Fructose, sugar in fruit, will not normally hurt you, but eaten at the wrong time or in the wrong combinations can create both digestive and metabolic problems. Therefore, what we are recommending is a *low-sugar diet.* Surprisingly, that cannot be achieved by simply putting away your sugar canister.

How can sugar, something that tastes so good and has been fed so readily to most of us since childhood by our most trusted person on earth, our mother, possibly be so bad for us? Aside from a few bad direct effects, such as dissolving our teeth, sugar largely acts as a stimulus in causing our pancreas gland to secrete one of the body's most powerful hormones, *insulin!*

Insulin has some good effects on our bodies, such as regulating our blood sugar level, but the bad effects caused by the overproduction of this megahormone are certainly impressive and will be described at length later. Succinctly, insulin causes our bodies to store excess sugar as fat. Insulin further inhibits the mobilization of previously stored fat, even if one is on a rather skimpy, but glucose-generating, diet. And, most significantly, insulin signals our livers to make the other big "C" word, cholesterol.

Now you might accept the first two and say, "Gee! That explains why I got fat or why I cannot get 'un-fat' even at a lower level of food consumption, but why should I buy this insulin-cholesterol connection?" Truth really is better than fiction, so let us relate an exchange between two of our authors.

After beginning to eat steak, lamb chops, cheese, eggs, and so on for the first time in fifteen years and seeing his cholesterol drop 21 percent and triglycerides by 50 percent, our CEO told his doctor (who also happens to be a heart surgeon) that the only thing that seemed to make sense was that insulin must be causing the liver to make cholesterol, because the main difference his low-sugar diet was causing was a lower average insulin level in his body. Our doctor paused about three seconds and said, "You know, you are right! When our borderline diabetics get to where they cannot control their diabetes with pills, diet, and exercise, and we have to give them insulin injections, we know the first major side effect will be that their cholesterol will become quite elevated, and as the insulin shots continue, the Type II diabetics will start getting more obese."

Our honest and perceptive doctor immediately recognized a frequently overlooked connection between insulin and cholesterol. In addition, our endocrinologist verified that his diabetic patients have significantly higher total cholesterol and triglycerides than the average population.

We are entering the twenty-first century and hardly anyone appreciates the insulin/cholesterol connection. Sounds crazy, but how many doctors or nutritionists have pushed that thought at you? Why have so many of our friends or patients who have gone on a low-sugar diet (not a *no*-sugar diet) lowered their cholesterol by an average of 15 percent without either exercise or pills? How could they have increased their fat intake and seen their cholesterol, triglyceride, and weight levels fall? It is the effect of lower average levels of *insulin* in their blood.

Carbohydrates are broken down to glucose (sugar) in our body, and this raises our blood sugar. Insulin is then secreted by the pancreas to lower our blood sugar, but in the process, insulin promotes the storage of fat and the elevation of cholesterol levels. Insulin also inhibits the breakdown of (loss of) previously stored fat. Not fancy, but fact. The charts in Figure 1 (page 16) "speak to this" in a beautifully simplistic fashion.

By the way, some of us are insulin resistant and

require large quantities of insulin to regulate our blood sugar levels. We have found nothing good about high average levels of insulin in our bodies. More on this later.

Let's review the essence of our "dietary lifestyle," which will be covered much more thoroughly in succeeding chapters. There are only a few things you cannot eat on this diet. They are the carbohydrates that cause an intense insulin secretion. You must virtually eliminate potatoes, corn, white rice, bread from refined flour, beets, carrots, and, of course, refined sugar, corn syrup, molasses, honey, sugared colas, and beer. Beyond that, you should eat fruit by itself. The list of foods allowed on the diet is extensive and will delight you by its length and variety.

Some of you will ask, "How much can I cheat on this diet?" The previous paragraph said to virtually eliminate refined sugars and certain carbohydrates. That means very little cheating. Get your sugar (glucose) through normal portions of all the acceptable carbohydrates listed in Chapter XI. Healthwise, this is the proper answer. Weightwise, some of you can cheat more than others and not gain weight, but if you have ever been significantly overweight, you had better cheat very infrequently.

Sound too simple? Well, it really is simple, but the "why" and "how" it works are somewhat more complex. When you understand the reasons the SUGAR BUSTERS! lifestyle works, you will be confident it is not another gimmicky diet, and you will tend to follow its guidelines more closely and enjoy the maximum benefits. So, please don't just jump to Chapter X, start the diet, and then not be able to tell anybody why you lost the weight and how you got that spring back in your step. Learn the benefits and enjoyment it can bring you for life—most probably, a longer life.

Are we the first to say certain food combinations are bad for you? No, but we think we have helped to verify why the specific way of eating we describe will be good for you, will help you lose weight without spending a penny on pills or spas, and will let you actually enjoy eating without the accompanying guilty conscience.

Calories are not the answer to weight gain or loss. The term *calorie* was first used by Lavoisier in the 1840s. Subsequently, a caloric theory developed that explained weight gain or loss. Although this theory was later proved flawed, nutritionists in the medical community ignored this correction.

We have been "hoaxed" for decades by the American nutrition industry, which either did not know better or had other obvious motives. The scientific data have been available in America for years for a logical researcher to come to this same conclusion. Americans alone spend $32 billion a year trying to lose weight, an additional $45.8 billion on medical costs directly related to problems caused by obesity, and $23 billion on time lost while away from the workplace because of the same problems (*Scientific American*, August 1996). Unfortunately, this is an incentive for some industries to ignore a way of eating that creates no profits. So, get ready: you have a lot of lifelong misinformation, misconceptions, and downright propaganda to overcome.

What motivates three doctors to tell you about something that will cost you only a few additional dollars each year on your grocery bill? Thank goodness, doctors are in the business to save lives. The message in this book can prolong lives and significantly improve the quality of life. The effects of a low-carbohydrate (sugar) diet will actually take patients away from many doctors.

What's wrong with losing weight in other ways? Some diets lead to partial starvation, the greatest negative effects being the depletion of many of the body's essential proteins, vitamins, and minerals, plus the misery you must endure of being constantly deprived of normal quantities of food. Of course, a whole industry is built on providing, at a price, vitamins and supplements in any quantity you might conceivably want. Ever taste a pill you really liked? Instead of having to swallow a pill, why not eat a plateful of savory meats and vegetables and lose weight in the process?

What a waste of money to spend $32 billion a year just to try and lose weight! Why not spend just a few dollars more on your regular food budget by replacing the most notorious insulin-stimulating carbohydrates, including starches, with other wholesome foods that you can buy at nearly any grocery store.

We have harped on insulin's bad effects, but we will now describe the benefits of another of the body's secretions. Glucagon, also shown on Figure 1 (page 16), is released from the pancreas into the bloodstream in significant quantities following the consumption of a protein-rich meal. Glucagon promotes the mobilization of previously stored fat; so, as you burn food reserves for your energy requirements between meals, high levels of glucagon will allow that energy to be derived from that spare tire around your waist. The glucagon chart also shows that, once the glucagon level is raised, it will remain elevated for quite some time so you can keep on burning that mobilized fat.

Remember, insulin *inhibits* the mobilization of previously stored fat. Because a high-protein meal does not stimulate significant amounts of insulin secretion, the fat mobilization inhibitor *is not* present, but a high level of glucagon, the fat mobilizer, *is* present.

The chart also shows that carbohydrate-rich meals actually suppress glucagon secretion. So, the stored-fat mobilizer is absent, but the hormone to promote storage, insulin, is present in significant amounts. When fat gets stored, we all know where it goes!

Ready for more good news? Following the pattern of eating we recommend can greatly relieve many common stomach maladies. One author went from Rolaids or Alka Seltzer twice a week to none (zero) for thirteen months while eating steak, lamb chops, cheese, and eggs for the first time in fifteen years. The only other alteration beyond a low-sugar diet was the substitution of red wine for other previously consumed spirits.

To drink or not to drink? You can find arguments both ways. But we believe, as do most American doctors, that, *if* you consume alcoholic beverages, the one that benefits you the most is red wine. Populations in countries with a higher relative consumption of red wine to other spirits definitely experience a lower incidence of cardiovascular disease.

One thing is for certain: alcohol consumption does not help you lose weight. However, with reasonably comfortable adjustments in eating habits, significant quantities of weight can be lost even with the continued consumption of modest amounts of alcohol like that contained in red wine.

How about exercise? Exercise is a definite plus

in overall body fitness and health, especially if done regularly and in moderate amounts. Nevertheless, a moderate amount of exercise will not significantly affect weight loss if you continue to eat foods that create a need for high levels of insulin in your bloodstream.

One author who has lost and kept off twenty pounds is not proud of the fact that he does not take the time to exercise, but he simply does not exercise (other than lifting his knife and fork!). So, the twenty-pound weight loss did not come from exercise or a low-calorie diet.

But, once again, we definitely believe exercise is good for you. In combination with the low-sugar diet we recommend, it should help with a general improvement in body weight control and health.

One word of caution: If you are a marathon runner or an exercise "fanatic," this diet is probably not for you. High levels of exercise require the foods that generate large quantities of glucose to feed your engine.

Does every person's body react to and process (metabolize) the identical meal in exactly the same way? No, but understanding the messages in this book will help you understand not only why, but also what, you can do to positively influence your own body's reaction to various foods and combinations of foods.

Some women have found it more difficult than men do to lose weight on any diet. This can be explained in part by the fact that shortly after birth a female's metabolic rate, on an age-adjusted basis, is approximately 10 percent lower than that of a male. Hormonal influences present in both premenopausal and postmenopausal women also may be responsible for difficulties in losing weight. Hormone therapy, in the form of either birth control pills or progesterone supplements, may further aggravate this problem. Chapter IX addresses in more detail the problems some women have experienced with weight loss because of hormonal intake.

Also, please be aware that even some of the most common over-the-counter preparations can cause fluid retention, increased appetite, and other changes that can lead to weight gain. However, all individuals, especially women, should be cautious about taking or discontinuing any type of medication without prior consultation with their physicians.

Although we specifically address sugar's causal and/or harmful effects on problems, such as weight gain, diabetes, and cardiovascular disease, we have not stressed the many other diseases or potentially harmful mental conditions influenced by consumption of large amounts of sugar. As we and others continue to cause or follow controlled research on sugar, other definitive observations will be forthcoming. But suffice it to say, with only the very harmful effects of overconsumption of sugar that we have documented in this book, it is likely that the list of sugar-induced problems will grow considerably.

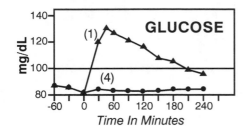

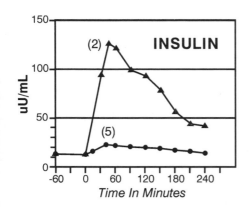

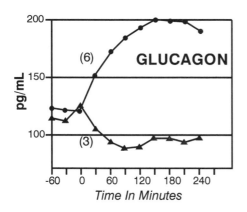

▲ High-carbohydrate meal
● High-protein meal

Figure 1.
Following a high-carbohydrate meal, glucose levels rise rapidly (1), stimulating the release of insulin (2), which promotes utilization of glucose but also signals the body to store fat and prevent the mobilization of previously stored fat. Glucagon secretion is suppressed by the high glucose level (3). A high-protein meal, however, causes only an imperceptible rise in blood glucose (4) and, consequently, a very small rise in insulin (5), but a significant increase in the glucagon level (6). Glucagon promotes the mobilization of previously stored fat.

Source: Modified from Wilson and Foster (1992).

II | A Brief History of Refined Sugar

Your ancestors did not do it, and neither did their dogs! In all the eons that our digestive systems were evolving, the world simply did not have refined sugar. A little honey for a few, yes. A little chew of the fibrous sugar cane for a few, yes. But for most of the world's inhabitants, no concentrated sugar at all—not in all those hundreds of thousands or millions of years.

Neither did those inhabitants have the luxury of being able to eat a combination of various classifications of food. They ate like all animals eat today (unless we force our pets to eat otherwise)—only one thing at a time, and that was in a completely unrefined form. They did not consume huge quantities of the types of hybridized or refined carbohydrates that would require large amounts of insulin secretion.

The pancreas gland was probably not called upon to secrete as much insulin in *one day* of an *entire lifetime* as it is called upon to secrete in nearly *every day* of a modern postinfant lifetime! For a visual example of how we have come from zero refined sugar intake in just the last fifteen centuries to our average daily consumption of refined sugar alone, see Figure 2 (page 19). And you are right; just think of how much more glucose (sugar) is generated with the carbohydrate and starch combinations of our "balanced American diet" that does not ever get picked up in the comparative statistics!

We have had refined sugar only for a mere blink of time in man's digestive evolution. Think about it. Is it any wonder that the incidence of diabetes and impaired glucose tolerance continues to get higher and higher? Maybe we simply wear out or exhaust our pancreas glands.

Where did the observations on sugar's ill effects originate? As refined sugar did not exist anywhere in the world until around A.D. 500, it must have been after that. The old holy books of the world's

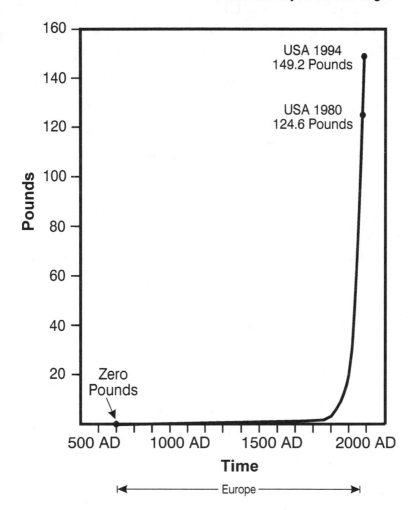

Figure 2.

Total refined sugar consumption per person per year.

Source: U.S. Department of Agriculture.

leading religions do not even mention sugar. Honey, yes; sugar, no. The early writers and historians did not have a word for it. If they had, they surely would have mentioned it prominently, as every society introduced to refined sugar has been immediately hooked on its delights and, unfortunately, also on its ill effects.

In more recent times, a physician in the seventeenth century, Dr. Thomas Willis (1647), wrote of his observation on diabetes and on some of the negative effects of sugar. Others wrote sparingly about it. If they wrote more, their works are not easily accessible.

In the early twentieth century, more attempts were made, with little effect, at alerting the world to the dangers of this refined substance. In 1976 William Dufty wrote *Sugar Blues*, which he said was inspired by the late famous actress Gloria Swanson, who recognized sugar's poisonous effects on both her mind and body.

Dufty's research, which summarized the observations of the earlier writers on sugar, pointed out sugar's profound negative effect on early armies, even entire nations, as it was introduced to them one by one. His research makes a strong (and logical) case that diabetes and other diseases grew significantly as refined sugar consumption increased.

Why have the early physicians' and anti-sugar crusaders' insights or observations never caught on? The refined-sugar lobby has been very powerful for a couple of centuries. The economic stakes in the sugar trade between nations were extremely high. Slavery even flourished because of it. Pro-sugar lobbying by sugar growers, cola manufacturers, and the packaged-food industry has been very effective in influencing our government. What politician wants to tell his or her constituents that they should no longer eat sugar?

Is it wrong to lobby *for* one's own product? No, but it is wrong to *minimize* the very serious side effects of refined-sugar consumption, such as causing a higher incidence of a very, very bad disease such as diabetes with all of its horrible effects on many organs of our bodies.

The main problem in society's ignorance of sugar's evil effects probably lies with our tendency to ignore what we do not want to hear.

There have been enough earlier crusaders for the sugar message to have caught on and been spread by the most effective form of communication, namely, word of mouth. It did not catch on; so, we simply must not have wanted to hear the message. Like alcoholics hooked on alcohol, we are hooked on sugar. We have said, "Just don't tell me that sugar is bad, too!"

Hearteningly, it took only a little over two years to see over 200,000 copies of the self-published version of this book sold and for it to build up a legion of successful followers. As the book was not advertised, the sales must have been by word of mouth. People simply needed a simple, straightforward explanation of how sugar consumption was really going to make them fat (and unhealthy).

If you are not in the frame of mind to give up most of your sugar consumption to improve your weight and health, a half-hearted effort, accompanied by constant cheating, will not allow this "diet" to work for you. Also, don't go overboard on adding extra helpings of the foods that you are allowed to eat, either!

There is some interesting information on average life span that might surprise you. The statistic that men's life expectancy has increased by 50 percent in the last century is accurate, but it is nearly all due to a tremendous decrease in infant and early childhood mortality. Middle-aged American men (+/-50 years old) only live eighteen months longer than they did in 1900, despite the availability of flu shots, penicillin for pneumonia, antibiotics, and general surgical technology, including early detection technology, transplant capability, and multiple life-support systems.

We also have refrigeration and improved packaging technology, which allows us to eat all varieties of food and minerals all year. And you can't go into any food store or drugstore without finding shelves and shelves of vitamins, minerals, and other supplements.

Why doesn't all this preventive medicine, year-round "balanced" diet availability, and life-support technology (that truly adds several years to many people's lives) result in more than an eighteen-month extension to a middle-aged man's life expectancy?

We believe the main culprit is the major change to refined foods and especially refined sugar. This has done to our entire population exactly what it did to the royalty of the last few centuries. Refined breads for the privileged, instead of raw or whole-grain breads, and consumption of large quantities of sugar and honey rapidly took their toll on the royalty by making them fat, giving them gout and apparently diabetes.

Just because we have everything in the world to eat doesn't mean we really eat better or even as well as most of our forefathers who ate in the fashion for which their digestive systems were designed. In fact, we believe that a middle-aged man's life expectancy has deteriorated—save and except for the medical wonders—and that his quality of life in his later years also has diminished on the average. The miraculous medical advances have been offset by the tremendous rise in sugar intake, as shown in Figure 2 (page 19).

It is quite logical that we should have added refined sugar to the priority list of things that are or may be "hazardous to your health" when you see the increase in disease caused by our huge consumption of refined sugar and certain other carbohydrates. Sugar just may be the number-one culprit in lowering quality of life and causing premature death. There certainly is enough evidence to bring us to that conclusion.

If the sugar-causes-disease message has not caught on yet, why do we think another book about it is worth the effort? Excess insulin is killing people prematurely, and even those who survive to an older age often have a greatly reduced quality of life. The importance of insulin has been ignored in the vast majority of nutritional and dietetic literature. The "insulin connection" needs to be understood and must be told over and over until it is appreciated.

You are the one to benefit from a low-sugar diet. One of the good old clichés is very applicable here: "Today is the first day of the rest of your life." Think about it.

Finally, the basic principles outlined in SUGAR BUSTERS! have been field-tested by the human digestive system throughout the eons. SUGAR BUSTERS! is unlike the new diet claims, health claims, and vitamin and supplement claims that are long on promise but short on field testing. These new claims are all too often proven to be false or ineffective after a few years of research. But every time a new claim gets widely publicized, someone or some industry makes a ton of money from the sales attached to it. In contrast, following the principles of the SUGAR BUSTERS! lifestyle costs nothing.

III | Myths

One of the first things we would like to do is dispel some of the concepts that have been around for so long that they are almost universally believed, even by the majority of doctors. The truth is that most doctors, dietitians, and other health professionals know very little about the complicated interplay of carbohydrates, fats, and proteins once these foods enter the body. This is an area where dogma has held sway or views have been conveniently retained for many years and only a few individuals have challenged these misconceptions. Let's examine some of these views more closely.

Calories and Weight Loss

What exactly is a calorie, and is it so important? A calorie is the amount of energy (heat) needed to raise 1 kilogram of water 1 degree Centigrade (from 15°C to 16°C). In other words, it is a measure of the amount of energy required to achieve a certain result. But how does this relate to the human body, and what does it mean for us?

If we were all internal combustion engines or boilers, then it would be easy to see how this concept would be important, because whatever amount of fuel went into our engine would come out as approximately an equivalent amount of energy. Theoretically, if one consumed an amount of food containing a certain number of calories, the body would have to expend this energy in a given period of time to remain calorie neutral. If not, the assumption has always been that the body will convert these excess calories into stored energy (fat!) that would be released at a later date when the body would need more energy than it had consumed. This has been the standard theory for decades, and, unfortunately, it has been well accepted by most nutritional professionals. In this model, as calorie requirements are exceeded by intake, fat will undoubtedly accumulate.

Most of these premises were based on research performed decades ago, research that was not verified by other investigators or subjected to the type of scrutiny and continued refinement that are usual with most scientific research performed today. Webb (1980) tabulated a number of overeating studies and accurately determined that energy intake (calories) is *not* sufficient to predict weight gain or loss in any given individual. Nevertheless, the caloric theory is widely accepted and has become deeply ingrained in the public psyche.

Fortunately, individuals have not evolved like engines, and caloric requirements and consumption never were meant to be in perfect equilibrium or so finely balanced that we should be overly concerned about small variations in either direction. In human beings, body weight is regulated by integrated and well-coordinated effects on food intake and energy expenditure, and the truth is that no one quite yet understands exactly how the body achieves this complex process. We now know that decreasing the amount of calories in the diet only leads to temporary weight loss, so there has to be a compensating process or another explanation.

Research has shown that, as we diet and lose weight, the body changes the amount of energy it expends. The body adjusts its energy requirements downward and thus needs to expend less energy to run itself (Leibel, Rosenbaum, and Hirsch, 1995). This presents a form of resistance to maintaining a reduced weight even while maintaining exactly the same low-calorie diet. This startling phenomenon accounts for the poor long-term results of most dietary treatments of obesity. We also get miserable eating less, and few of us will fight that situation for the remainder of our lives; we will ultimately give in to one of life's greatest pleasures, which is eating in normal quantities.

Our view is that calories per se are not as important as the types of food we eat, how we eat them, and what metabolic processes control their assimilation. What we do know is that normal, even significant, amounts of the proper types of food can be consumed for indefinite periods without causing weight gain!

Fats and Weight Gain

Because fats provide more calories per gram (9) than either carbohydrates or protein (4), it has always been a popular myth that fats are bad. This has been driven in large part by the calorie-counting myth, that is, fat grams result in more calories than carbohydrate grams; therefore, eating fewer fat and more carbohydrate grams will result in consuming fewer overall calories and a healthier diet. This reasoning has given tremendous impetus to the consumption of certain types of carbohydrates, such as pasta, potatoes, and rice. This trend has now reached unprecedented proportions in this country with the current pasta craze.

The fact is that fats, in and of themselves, do not necessarily cause weight gain. Moreover, fats are vitally important to the body by providing essential elements, such as fatty acids, many vitamins, and hormones important for metabolic processes. It is true that many of us consume more fat than we need, but this is largely due to the fact that fats are present in so many food items that have become popular in this country: fast foods such as doughnuts, fried chicken, or french fries. Therefore, although consumption of a reasonable amount of fat is healthy, we agree that it is generally necessary to trim the large amount of saturated fats consumed in the normal American diet.

As the ingestion of fats as well as carbohydrates may lead to changes in cholesterol, it is very important to point out that some fats lower cholesterol and others raise it. For instance, monounsaturated fatty acids contained in foods such as olive oil, canola oil, peanut oil, and pecans may in fact be helpful for patients with coronary artery disease or with a high risk of developing coronary disease.

Reliable studies have confirmed that low rates of coronary artery disease occur in Mediterranean countries where the population consumes a large percentage of their calories as these monounsaturated fats, primarily in the form of olive oil. Other studies show similar beneficial effects for walnuts and almonds, both rich in monounsaturated fats (O'Keefe, Lavier, and McCallister, 1995).

However, saturated fats and many polyunsaturated fats are believed to lead to an increased risk for development of coronary disease. In a recent study where patients were randomly assigned to receive a Mediterranean-type diet that was high in vegetables, fresh fruit, whole grains, and olive oil compared to a standard diet, there was a 79 percent decrease in major cardiovascular events after twenty-seven months in the Mediterranean group (deLorgeril, Mamelle, and Salem, 1993). Yet the standard diet recommended for patients with or at risk for coronary disease is to consume 70 percent to 85 percent of calories from carbohydrates with very low amounts of fat and protein! It is very possible that this may be just the wrong recommendation for many patients because such a diet can actually increase triglyceride levels and decrease high-density lipoprotein (HDL) cholesterol, the "protective" cholesterol (the higher the HDL, the better).

Another class of fats that may be beneficial for heart disease is the omega-3-polyunsaturated acids, or fish oils. These oils decrease triglyceride levels and decrease the stickiness of platelets in the bloodstream. Elevated triglycerides, or "sticky" platelets, usually contribute to, or even cause, the start of arteriosclerosis.

Our view then is that not all fats are the same

and they should not be considered as having the same effect when eaten. Many, in fact, are actually good for you and are covered further in Chapter IV.

Cholesterol

A closely related myth is the cholesterol story. Cholesterol was not a major consideration until the early 1970s. At that time guidelines were first issued in the United States warning against the dangers of butter, eggs, lard, and other animal fats. This produced the current trend of classifying foods as either healthy or unhealthy.

The relationship between fats (triglycerides), cholesterol, and heart disease was presented in the "seven countries' study." This study recommended that fat intake be reduced to 30 percent of total energy intake. However, the study revealed that in the Netherlands' population, the percentage of energy derived from fat was 48 percent, but their life expectancy was one of the highest in Europe!

Similarly, in Crete, fat consumption was 40

percent of total energy intake, but the incidence of heart disease was one of the lowest in Europe. These inconsistencies have never been satisfactorily explained, although we agree that very high cholesterol levels (more than 300 mg/dL*) are significantly related to coronary artery disease (Artaud-Wild, Connor, Sexton, and Connor, 1993).

Furthermore, the clinical studies directed at lowering lipids, including cholesterol, have shown no consistent decrease in death rates in spite of success in lowering cholesterol. In some studies more than half the patients with coronary disease had cholesterol levels below 200 mg/dL (Anderson, Castelli, and Levy, 1987). The message is in most instances that total cholesterol alone is not a reliable indicator for the risk of cardiovascular disease.

Alcohol Is Always Bad for You

We all have heard over and over how fattening alcohol is, but this is only partially true. Compared

---

*mg/dL (milligrams per deciliter) is the laboratory scale for measuring blood cholesterol levels.

to many other carbohydrates, alcohol is far less fattening. For instance, a glass of wine has fewer calories than a slice of white bread. The body generally utilizes the alcohol as an immediate source of energy. While doing this, the body will not burn any energy from body reserves (fat!). The conclusion here is that alcohol would prevent any weight loss. But this could be said of anything that delivers a significant amount of energy to our bodies.

It appears that this negative effect is most pronounced when alcohol is taken on an empty stomach. This effect is minimized if you drink alcohol after first putting some food into your stomach, particularly foods composed of protein or lipids that do not allow the alcohol to reach the small intestine so rapidly, where it then can be quickly absorbed into the bloodstream.

Some forms of alcohol are worse than others. For instance, beer has a high content of maltose, a carbohydrate that causes a rapid increase in blood sugar, which makes it a type of drink that needs to be avoided. Likewise, all after-dinner type drinks and liqueurs have a high content of sugar and should be avoided.

Wine is perhaps the most acceptable form of alcohol. It has been shown that the death rate from heart attacks is lowest in countries where wine is habitually consumed, such as France, Italy, and Spain.

The truth is that alcohol in moderation—and particularly red wine—when taken after the ingestion of protein or lipids (like a piece of meat or cheese) will not be as harmful as you would be led to believe and can actually be beneficial in delaying the onset of or reducing the advancement of arteriosclerosis. Excessive alcohol consumption, however, usually causes harmful effects that far outweigh any of its benefits.

IV | Digestion and Metabolism

The digestion and metabolism of the foods we eat are the keys to success in maintaining good nutrition and normal body weight. Because "we are what we eat," this is an important chapter for the proper understanding of our diet concept. It will provide you with a basic understanding of these processes so that you can maximize your gains in achieving these goals. This book is being written for a broad audience, including health care professionals, so we will use some technical terms from time to time. As mentioned, if you come to a term you do not understand, please look it up in the Layman's Glossary.

Digestion

Digestion encompasses the entire process from the time food is eaten until it is finally absorbed by the intestinal cells and sent on its way to the liver for metabolism. The most important aspect of digestion is the breakdown of proteins, fats, and carbohydrates into succcssively smaller units that can then be absorbed into the bloodstream and lymphatics to be used by the body in different ways.

Before any of this can happen, an integral part of the digestive process is the mixing and the churning (much like a concrete mixer) that occurs in the stomach. This process allows foods to be softened and mixed with fluid and be subjected to the initial phases of digestion. This mixing finally culminates in the gradual emptying of material from the stomach into the small intestine. Liquids empty from the stomach fairly quickly, within minutes, but solids empty much more slowly. The time that it takes for half of the stomach's solid contents to empty is somewhere between thirty and sixty minutes.

Smaller solid particles empty before larger ones

in a very orderly, sequential fashion. The last solids to empty are fiber or indigestible solids, such as those found in leafy vegetables. When your mother advised, "Chew your food well," she was instinctively telling you the right thing to do because the smaller the particles, the more quickly the food would clear your stomach and, perhaps, avoid that uncomfortable feeling of fullness or the onset of indigestion.

Stomach emptying can be delayed by many external factors, including the types of foods eaten. A meal containing a large amount of fat can significantly delay stomach emptying, as can the drinking of large amounts of alcohol prior to, or with, the meal. Slow or delayed stomach emptying can then lead to the reflux of stomach contents—by this time usually very acidic—into the lower esophagus, causing heartburn, chest discomfort, fullness, and even nausea and vomiting. Many of us can recall these problems after a late evening of dining and drinking and going to bed with a full stomach!

As this stomach mix is gradually emptied into the small intestine, the breakdown of foods for absorption by our bodies begins in earnest. In the first part of the small intestine, called the duodenum, bile from the gallbladder and enzymes from the pancreas mix with the stomach contents and speed the breakdown of the different foods into smaller and smaller units. This mix moves farther down the small intestine where absorption takes place by the cells lining the intestine.

It is important to point out that the mixing of certain foods can have tremendous implications later on as these smaller units become absorbed. For instance, eating foods containing a modest amount of insoluble fiber can affect the rate of digestion and absorption of carbohydrates, thus causing these carbohydrates to have a much lower insulin-stimulating effect than if eaten by themselves. This would obviously be a good thing for the body.

Fruits eaten by themselves also are digested and absorbed at better rates than if eaten together with other carbohydrates and fats. The negative effect that eating fruits at the wrong time can have on the other foods in the digestive process is covered in Chapter XII.

Metabolism

To *metabolize* essentially means "to change" and it entails the many processes that transform the nutrients in food to chemical substances that can be used by our bodies. The entire process is obviously quite complex. Metabolic rates often vary from person to person. This means that weight gain or loss for two people on the identical diet can vary considerably.

Although the process is complex, you should know that the liver plays the central role in the metabolism of foods, including alcohol, and in the metabolism of the majority of medications. So it is easy to see the importance of the liver in our nutritional well-being, and it behooves us all to take very good care of it because medical science cannot yet duplicate its functions. When the liver goes, it is "Adios, amigo!"

Now let's talk about what types of food get metabolized for use by our bodies. Everything we eat is either carbohydrates, which are broken down to simple sugar, 80 percent glucose and the rest fructose or galactose depending on whether we have had fruit or dairy products; proteins, which are broken down to amino acids; fats, which are broken down to triglycerides; and fiber, which is cellulose and cannot be broken down further. Of these four substances, only three are absorbed from our digestive tracts: sugars, amino acids, and triglycerides.

Carbohydrates

Carbohydrates can be found in both plant and animal food sources. The overwhelming majority of the carbohydrates we eat are in the form of sugars and starches. Carbohydrates can be classified as simple sugars or more complex sugars, such as starch.

All carbohydrates absorbed by the body are eventually converted to glucose. Glucose is the body's main fuel, much like the gasoline that is put in a car. Glucose is either used immediately to provide energy or stored in the form of glycogen in the liver and in muscle to be utilized later. Any remaining glucose then is stored as fat.

In understanding the metabolism of carbohydrates and how this relates to our recommendations for good nutrition and weight loss, it is very important to think of carbohydrates in terms of how much of a peak or rise of glucose they can cause within the body when eaten. This can be more simply called the glycemic potential, which varies for different types of carbohydrates and in more scientific terms can be defined as the glycemic index. The glycemic index graph in Figure 3 (page 45) simply reflects the area under the curve representing the rise in blood sugar over a given time. Glucose has been assigned a relative value of 100 as its glycemic index, and the values of other carbohydrates are simply related to this level. Some substances actually have a higher glycemic potential than glucose! You will see more on the importance of a carbohydrate's glycemic potential later.

When the blood glucose level drops lower than it should be, glycogen, which is glucose in its stored form in the body, is broken down into glucose to raise the level of glucose and maintain a normal blood sugar level.

Carbohydrates, such as starches, which have a more complex structure, can, contrary to some commonly held beliefs, be digested and absorbed nearly as fast as the more simple carbohydrates, such as table sugar. When a carbohydrate is eaten, there is a rise in the level of blood glucose commensurate with the type and amount of carbohy-

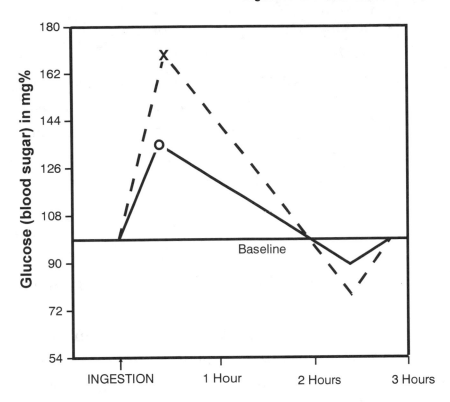

Figure 3.
Glycemic index graph.

X=High-glycemic carbohydrate; O=Low-glycemic carbohydrate.

drate ingested (i.e., higher for sugar, lower for fresh fruit). This rise in blood sugar (glucose) is then followed by the release of insulin, which causes a fall in the level of glucose primarily as it is driven into the cells of the body where it can be utilized as instant fuel or stored mainly as fat. Following this, the glucose level returns to its normal baseline.

Proteins

Proteins, the sources of which are meats, nuts, dairy products, and some vegetables, are made of subunits called amino acids. These amino acids are released from the protein by the action of enzymes secreted by the pancreas. Without these enzymes, protein molecules would not be absorbed because they are too large and complex to enter the bloodstream. Fortunately, in cases where pancreatic enzymes are missing, they can be provided in capsule form that can be taken with meals to aid the digestive process.

An average adult should consume per day *at least* one gram of protein for each kilogram (2.2 pounds) of weight, or somewhere between 55 and

70 grams (2 to 2.5 ounces) for the average man or woman.

Because there are both animal and vegetable sources of proteins and neither of these sources provides all of the amino acids that the body needs, a diet should be well balanced to provide both sources of protein.

Once proteins have been broken down into amino acids, they can be absorbed from the intestine and metabolized by the liver. Then, in general, amino acids can either be used by the body as the basic building blocks of all proteins, which make up all cells, hormones, and neurotransmitters (substances that relay signals in the nervous system), or amino acids can be converted into glucose, or sugar, by the liver through a process called *gluconeogenesis*, which is the manufacture of glucose from noncarbohydrate food sources, such as protein. The body's ability to manufacture its own glucose is important for maintaining normal energy requirements during periods of low-carbohydrate consumption, as glucose is the main fuel the body uses to meet its energy requirements.

Fats

Fats, or lipids, are complex molecules composed of fatty acids and are derived from both animal and vegetable origins. Fats must be digested through the actions of pancreatic enzymes called lipases; otherwise, they cannot enter the body to any great extent and are passed in the stool. Even after fats are broken down into subunits, most of these remain insoluble in water and require a special type of absorption. Bile from the liver, which is stored in the gallbladder, plays a very important role in this absorption of fats by emulsifying or dissolving them. This is akin to using soap or any detergent to help in dissolving an oily substance. Without this process, fat subunits would be too large to enter the bloodstream from the intestine.

Some individuals who lack pancreatic enzymes must take enzymes with their food. Fats are absorbed through the intestinal tract as glycerols and are reconstituted while still in the intestinal wall as triglycerides that then enter the lymphatic system where these fats can be used by all the body's cells.

Cells use fat as fuel for energy production, as an important component of cell structures, and as a source of many essential substances manufactured by cells. An important function of fat that no one likes to think of is to provide insulation in the form of a layer of fat immediately underneath the skin. This should be only a thin layer, however, and it is almost always a source of constant restructuring in modern man and woman's attempts to control weight and body shape.

Cholesterol is not what most people think. Contrary to common belief, cholesterol is not a fat and has nothing to do with saturated fats. It is a compound belonging to a family of substances called *sterols*. Cholesterol can combine with fat as it circulates in the bloodstream to be distributed to all cells. Cholesterol is a vital substance in the formation of steroids, bile acids, hormones, and other substances.

Because cholesterol is so important, the body must provide a constant supply of cholesterol to the cells. Therefore, the body not only takes in cholesterol from food but also manufactures it, primarily in the liver. The liver can provide enough cholesterol to meet the body's needs even if a person were to take in no cholesterol in food! Cholesterol manufactured in the liver circulates as lipoproteins for delivery to the cells. It is during this circulation in the bloodstream that cholesterol can be deposited on major arterial walls, especially at points of irritation, roughness, or small breaks in the lining of these vessels. This is the process referred to as *arteriosclerosis*, and it is the underlying process leading to coronary heart disease and in some cases hypertension (high blood pressure).

Now you know how your digestive system works and some of the things that help or hinder its efficiency. We keep mentioning and hinting at the importance of insulin. The next chapter is dedicated to helping you better understand the insulin connection.

V | Insulin

You may ask, "Why do I want to know more about insulin? It is just another seven-letter hormone." Insulin is the maestro, the conductor, the chief. It is the CEO of metabolism. We must understand the actions of insulin to understand why the diet works.

Ready for some additional technical, but hopefully interesting, information? Banting and Best discovered insulin in 1921. This hormone is manufactured and secreted by the beta cells of the pancreas. The human pancreas stores about two hundred units of insulin. Normal people secrete about twenty-five to thirty units of insulin daily. Insulin is like a broom. It sweeps glucose, amino acids, and free fatty acids into cells where potential energy is stored as fat and glycogen to be used later.

In normal individuals, blood sugar levels do not vary much because of the harmonious and compensating hormonal actions of insulin and glucagon. Insulin is the only hormone that can prevent sugar (glucose) from rising to dangerously high levels. Glucagon, also secreted by the pancreas, prevents the blood sugar from falling too low (to hypoglycemic levels).

Whereas insulin has been referred to as the hormone of feasting, glucagon is the hormone of fasting (or starvation). The main role of glucagon in humans appears to be the prevention of hypoglycemia (low blood glucose or blood sugar) by causing the normal breakdown of glycogen in the liver to form glucose. It also causes gluconeogenesis, which is the conversion of muscle protein to blood sugar.

Gluconeogenesis can occur during periods of starvation or excessive exercise. During the first twenty-four hours of fasting, glycogen in the liver is utilized, and then the body will begin using up muscle proteins. Glucagon secretion is stimulated by hypoglycemia, fasting, and also by the ingestion of a protein-rich meal.

Individuals can survive without glucagon, as in cases where the pancreas, which is the only known source of glucagon and insulin, is removed. A person must have insulin to survive, and this can be accomplished through insulin injections. Of course, removing the pancreas causes diabetes, often with wide swings in the blood sugar levels. Insulin given by injections is not as efficient in providing a continuous supply in exactly the right amount as is the pancreas.

After a person eats carbohydrates, the digestive enzymes break down the food. The blood in the intestines, having absorbed these simplified food substances, now has an elevated glucose level. This stimulates the release of insulin. As we have previously learned, insulin causes the storage of fat. When the blood sugar level falls too low, glucagon is secreted, which mobilizes stored fat into glucose, which raises blood sugar back to its normal level.

Glucose is the major stimulus for insulin secretion. Fructose, a sugar from fruits, and amino acids (proteins) from meats, cause a significant release of insulin only in the presence of previously elevated blood sugar. The overweight person probably has increased insulin production because of excessive stimulation of the pancreas through overeating and the development of, or genetic tendency toward, insulin resistance.

The increased insulin level then promotes the storage of sugar as glycogen in both the liver and muscle. After proteins and fats are ingested, insulin promotes the storage of protein in muscle and fat in fat cells as triglycerides. Insulin also prevents the breakdown of glycogen and triglycerides (fat). No wonder it is difficult to lose weight in the presence of elevated insulin levels.

Scientific literature documents that even low levels of circulating insulin inhibit fat breakdown (Kahn and Weir, 1994). The metabolic pathways involving insulin are exquisitely sensitive in causing the storage of fat and inhibiting its breakdown for use by the body.

Insulin further activates an enzyme, lipoprotein lipase (enzymes are proteins that speed up metabolic actions), that promotes the removal of triglycerides from the bloodstream and their deposition in fat cells. Insulin also inhibits hormone-sensitive lipase (another enzyme) that breaks down stored fats. The net result of these two activities is an increase in stored fat that results in weight gain and an increase of abdominal girth.

Also adding to fat storage is the conversion of some of the sugar present in the blood. A percentage of the blood sugar is taken up by fat cells and, under the influence of our old friend insulin, is converted to still more fat. For our scientific readers, this involves glycerol 3-phosphate and free fatty acids. Insulin is a major deterrent to fat breakdown and a major facilitator of fat storage.

Insulin resistance is a condition of decreased responsiveness to insulin wherein the fat cells, liver cells, and muscle cells have become insensitive to normal levels of circulating insulin. Usually a small burst of insulin will lower blood sugar. However, in an insulin-resistant individual, this does not occur, and more insulin is required to do the job.

Obesity is the most common result of insulin resistance. Another frequently seen result of insulin resistance is Type II diabetes (non-insulin-dependent diabetes). In most Type II diabetics the circulating insulin levels and blood sugars are elevated, as are the blood cholesterol levels.

Obese individuals without diabetes usually have elevated insulin levels with normal blood sugar levels. Unfortunately, the obese person with an elevated insulin level may be on his way to developing diabetes. The pancreas may simply become exhausted from constant stimulation by glucose (sugar) and finally fail, resulting in diabetes. Diabetes is discussed specifically in Chapter VI.

Insulin promotes the storage of all food groups: glucose (carbohydrates), amino acids (proteins), and triglycerides (fats). These stored foods are available for use as an energy source later in a fasting state or simply between meals. The fall in insulin levels during fasting allows the breakdown of stored fat and stored sugar (glycogen). Fats and glycogen are then used as energy sources between meals.

As mentioned, obese people have elevated insulin levels in both the fasting and fed states. Lipoprotein lipase levels also are elevated in the obese. The enzyme, lipoprotein lipase, is important in the storage of fat. You now can see that obese individuals are metabolically ready at all times to store whatever they eat.

Again, it's no wonder that the obese person with an elevated insulin level has a hard time losing weight. But think of the benefits of a diet for this very same person that requires the presence of very little insulin in the system. We are now gaining on the answer to how to lose weight and improve our blood chemistry at the same time.

Syndrome X, described by Dr. G. M. Reaven, is a combination of two or more of the following conditions: insulin resistance with resulting elevated insulin levels, elevated lipids (especially triglycerides), obesity, coronary artery disease, and hypertension. Insulin resistance probably is the most important part of this syndrome because in fact it often causes the other problems to occur. A significant number of patients with Syndrome X develop coronary artery disease and experience an increased number of fatal heart attacks (O'Keefe, Lanier, and McCallister, 1995).

How about some good news? Fifty percent or more of insulin resistance can be reduced or even reversed as insulin resistance does not totally depend on our inherited genes. How can we decrease insulin levels or reduce insulin resistance? You are right! It's the SUGAR BUSTERS! way of eating. First, we must eat less of the particularly insulin-stimulating carbohydrates. This helps with weight loss and, combined with exercise and smoking cessation, provides major nonmedical ways to accomplish this reduction of circulating insulin. Therefore, by lowering the insulin levels and decreasing insulin resistance, the incidence of obesity and probably the progression of heart disease will decrease.

Many people with coronary artery disease have similar body shapes. They are fatter in the abdomen, have beer bellies, and are thinner in the hips and buttocks. This is called central obesity (apple shape). Individuals with diabetes and insulin resistance have similar apple shapes, as opposed to pear shapes, where the fat is distributed in the hips and buttocks.

Dr. Wolever and coworkers in 1992 studied the benefits of a low-glycemic index diet in overweight non-insulin-dependent diabetics. They found a 7 percent drop in cholesterol after only six weeks. Dr. Jenkins (1987) studied a low-glycemic (low-sugar) diet fed to normal males. After two weeks the men's cholesterol dropped an average of 15 percent, and insulin secretion dropped an amazing 32 percent!

After ingestion of 50 to 100 grams of glucose during a high-sugar meal, insulin levels usually become very elevated and can remain elevated for several hours. Eating high-carbohydrate (high-glycemic) meals three times a day and at bedtime can cause insulin to be elevated for eighteen out of twenty-four hours. The pancreas needs a rest, and so do fat cells. Imagine insulin pushing fat into cells eighteen hours a day. Only a few hours a day would be left for fat breakdown and fat loss. Fat would tend to accumulate at essentially all other times, resulting in you know what going you know where!

Understanding insulin and metabolism will now enable us to follow a healthier diet. As mentioned, not all carbohydrates are equal in their ability to stimulate insulin release. Carbohydrates that stimulate the most insulin secretion are called high-glycemic carbohydrates. Conversely, low-glycemic carbohydrates do not stimulate as much insulin secretion.

Because we have learned that we need to dodge the carbohydrates with the high glycemic indexes, we are now going to provide you with some additional glycemic index formation. In 1981 Dr. David Jenkins published an article on the glycemic indexes of foods in the *American Journal of Clinical Nutrition*. He and others have since provided many additional measurements on the glycemic indexes of certain carbohydrates. Figure 4 (pages 61–65) lists the glycemic indexes for many of our most commonly consumed carbohydrates.

Figure 4.
Glycemic index

(Compiled from multiple glycemic studies. Some numbers are slightly rounded.)

Grains, Breads, and Cereals
It is very difficult to find breakfast cereals that are processed without the addition of one or more of the sugars. Read the labels closely and go with those that have very little or no added sugar, the highest fiber or bran content, and the least processing of the grain. Also avoid corn-based cereals.

Of the pastas, stone-ground whole-grain pasta would be the best. Next best would be a stone-ground whole-wheat pasta.

HIGH			
White bread	95	Corn chips	75
French bread	95	Graham crackers	75
Instant rice	90	Regular crackers	75
White pretzels	85	White bagel	75
Rice cakes	80	Total cereal	75
Rice Crispies	80	Cheerios, white flour	75
Corn	75	Puffed wheat	75

Cornflakes	70–75	Brown rice	55
Croissant	70	Oatmeal	55
Corn meal	70	Special K	55
White rice	70	Muesli, no sugar added	55
Taco shells	70	Whole-grain	
Cream of Wheat	70	pumpernickel	50
Shredded wheat,		Cracked-wheat	
white flour	70	bulgur bread	50
Melba toast	70	High % cracked-wheat	
Millet	70	bread	50
Grape Nuts	65	Whole rice	50
Whole-wheat crackers	65	Oat and bran bread	50
Nutri-grain cereal	65	Sponge cake	45
Stoned Wheat Thins	65	Pita bread, stone-ground	45
Regular pasta	65	Wheat grain	45
Couscous	60	Barley grain	45
Basmati rice	60	Whole-grain pasta	45
Spaghetti, white	60	All Bran, no sugar added	45
		Whole-meal spaghetti	40
MODERATE			
Pita bread, regular	55	**LOW**	
Rye sourdough	55	Rye grain	35
Wild rice	55		

Vegetables

Most vegetables are very good in providing much of the natural "carbohydrate sugar" we definitely should include in our daily diets. A few, however, do stimulate excessive insulin secretion and they should be avoided. For a more complete listing of the acceptable vegetables, please refer to Figure 10 (pages 123–124).

HIGH		LOW	
Baked potato	95	Dried beans, lentils	30–40
Parsnips	95	Pinto beans	40
Carrots	85	Green beans	40
French fries	80	Chick peas	35
Beets	75	Lima beans	30
		Black beans	30
MODERATE		Butter beans	30
Sweet potatoes	55	Kidney beans	30
Yams	50	Soy beans	15
Green peas	45	Green vegetables (fig. 10,	
Black-eyed peas	40	pages 123–124)	0–15

Fruits

Fruits are a great source of sugar because they generally have a moderate to low insulin-stimulating effect and also provide vitamins necessary to good health. As explained, however, fruits are handled best by our digestive system if consumed alone. While not individually listed, fruit juices generally have a modestly higher glycemic index than the whole fruit itself.

HIGH			
		Peaches	40
Watermelon	70	Plums	40
Pineapple	65	Apples	40
Raisins	65	Oranges	40
Ripe bananas	60		
		LOW	
MODERATE		Apricots, dried	30
Mango	50	Grapefruit	25
Kiwi	50	Cherries	25
Grapes	50	Tomatoes	15
Plantain banana	45	Apricots, fresh	10
Pears	45		

Dairy Products

Dairy products also provide many of the vitamins necessary to good health. Furthermore, except for dairy products with added sugar, they all possess a moderate to low insulin-stimulating effect. But

please don't overdo the amount of fat consumed
through dairy products.

HIGH		Milk, whole	>30
Ice cream, premium	60	Milk, skimmed	<30
		Yogurt, plain, no sugar	15
MODERATE			
Yogurt, with added fruit	35		

Miscellaneous

HIGH		Popcorn	55
Maltose (as in beer)	105		
Glucose	100	LOW	
Pretzels	80	Nuts	15–30
Honey	75	Peanuts	15
Refined sugar	75		

The glycemic index is a method of classifying foods according to their glycemic effects or, simply stated, by the ability of a specific food to raise our blood sugar levels. As the blood sugar rises, the demand for insulin also rises. Knowledge of the glycemic index is a key to understanding the SUGAR BUSTERS! diet concept. Unfortunately, information on the glycemic index is not available on the labels listing a food's contents. The form of foods we eat, such as whole-grain versus refined flour, the size of the particles of food, the biologic nature of the starch, and the processing of foods all play a significant role in the physiologic properties of foods. These properties affect the glycemic index. In this chapter we have summarized what we have found on the glycemic indexes of common foods. If a specific common food is not covered, we simply could not find it.

As seen in Figure 4 (pages 61–65), the glycemic index is a number related to the total area under the curve illustrating the rise in blood glucose (sugars) over time. A high-glycemic index carbohydrate causes a greater level of blood sugar than does the same amount of a low-glycemic index

carbohydrate. Consuming a high-glycemic carbohydrate also can result subsequently in hypoglycemia, a lower-than-normal blood sugar through
excessive insulin secretion. This is discussed in
Chapter VII.

The higher the level of blood sugar, the more
insulin needs to be secreted by the pancreas to
utilize or remove the glucose and bring the blood
sugar level back to normal. This insulinemia, or
high blood insulin level, we feel is harmful, leading to metabolic changes and problems.

The medical and nutrition literature is beginning to contain many reports listing the glycemic
index for various types of carbohydrates, as measured in both healthy adults and diabetics. Test
foods are fed to subjects who also are fed on another day a known quantity of glucose or white
bread that serves as the standard against which
the various foods are compared. Blood sugar levels
are then measured at specific timed intervals up
to two hours after the test food is eaten, and the
resulting values are plotted on a graph (Figure 3,
page 45). The area under the glycemic response
curve for each food is then expressed as a percent

of the response obtained from glucose or white bread. Several measurements of glycemic reactions to the same food are averaged to obtain the glycemic index for that particular test food.

We feel that a very important determinant of the glycemic index is the particle size and form in which a carbohydrate comes packaged by nature. Cracked grains produce a lower glycemic index than coarse flour, which in turn produces a lower glycemic index than finely milled flour (Figure 5, page 69). The lowest glycemic indexes are associated with the whole grains (Heator et al., 1988). It is no surprise that whole or cracked grains produce the lowest insulin response. When whole, rolled, or finely milled oats (oatmeal) are compared, the whole oats have the lowest glycemic index.

While particle size significantly affects the glycemic index, data show that the form of the carbohydrate also contributes to glycemic differences. For example, when starches are cooked, they become gelatinized. The particles or granules swell because of the heat and water absorbed during cooking. This leads to a rupture of the granule, exposing the individual starch molecules, thus increasing the susceptibility of the starch to en-

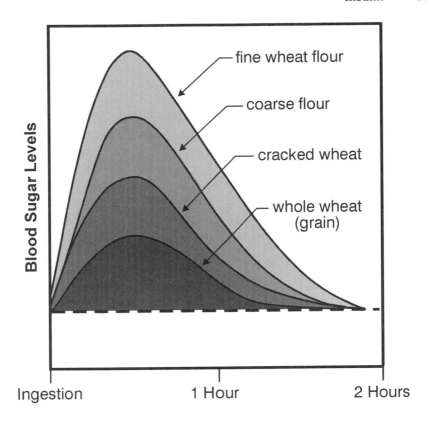

The larger the particle size, the lower the glycemic index

Figure 5.
Effects of processing grain

zymatic digestion. This leads to a more rapid absorption through the walls of the small intestine (Chapter IV). When a carbohydrate is absorbed quickly, it stimulates more insulin than the same amount of a more slowly absorbed carbohydrate. Medical studies have shown that processing wheat products leads to a higher glycemic index for these foods. Modern food processing may include puffing, thermal extrusion, intense mechanical treatments, and canning, all of which alter the foods to a considerable degree. Generally, products with the least degree of processing have the lowest glycemic index. Therefore, the more processing a carbohydrate such as rice, corn, or wheat has been subjected to, the higher its glycemic index.

We have now developed a more extensive glycemic index table for a variety of carbohydrate-containing foods that we hope will be useful when selecting food items and preparing meals. Figure 4 (pages 61–65) illustrates the glycemic index of many carbohydrates and gives you information on foods in the high-, moderate-, and low-glycemic index categories. These categories offer you a simple and general approach to eating. Unfortunately, some foods are not listed. In these instances, we recommend that you attempt to compare the unlisted item to a closely related item and use that value. For instance, the glycemic index for a white potato is probably very similar for an Idaho or Irish potato.

Reading labels on essentially all processed or packaged foods is important. Most of the sugar is added during the processing or packaging. If an ingredient, such as sugar or a sugar derivative, is not specifically broken out and listed in the grams column, you can sometimes estimate the amount by remembering that ingredients are (supposed to be) listed in the order of their abundance. For instance if a sugar derivative, such as maltodextrin, is listed first or second, don't use that product unless it is in extremely small amounts.

Grains, Breads, and Cereals

As mentioned, it is important to read the labels of breads, cereals, or pasta to get an idea of what types of grains and how much processing have been used in preparation of these foods. Whole wheat sounds good, but can be very misleading. It can apply to breads consisting mainly of the whole grain, which are very acceptable, but also to breads made from highly refined flour, which often are referred to as whole wheat, but possibly retain none of the grain husk. *Whole-grain* breads or cereals have as their main ingredient the whole or cracked grain. *Whole meal* refers to a grain product that has been partially processed. But whole meal is better than finely milled or highly refined flour that has been stripped of most of its fiber. We recommend whole-grain breads that have the intact or cracked kernel as much as possible. The higher the percentage (50 percent or more), the better. So, read the labels on breads. Finding the grain percentages listed on the labels is not very common in the United States, however.

Another problem is enriching, which usually means the grain initially has been so highly processed that even the vitamins and minerals have been stripped out and must be replaced (enriched). Sometimes labels contain all the information needed; unfortunately, in many instances they do not. If all else fails, remember what the grandmother of one of our friends said: "The whiter the bread, the quicker you're dead!" Figure 4 (pages 61–65) lists the glycemic indexes for many of our most commonly consumed carbohydrates.

VI | Why SUGAR BUSTERS! Works for Diabetics

This chapter should be read by everyone, not just those individuals with diabetes. We all know friends or relatives with diabetes. After you read this book and particularly this chapter, you will be able to give those diabetics some intriguing advice that will make them go back to their doctors and begin eating in a way that will reduce their blood sugar levels and, thereby, their need for as much insulin or oral medications.

The two main categories of diabetes are *insulin-dependent*, or *Type I*, diabetes and *non-insulin-dependent*, or *Type II*, diabetes, although many Type II diabetics ultimately become dependent on orally administered medication or injections of insulin to control their blood sugars. Another less common type of diabetes occurs during pregnancy.

This is referred to as *gestational diabetes*, which we will discuss later in this chapter.

Over 90 percent of all patients with diabetes have Type II diabetes. Type I diabetics are generally younger, thinner, and require insulin injections. Type II diabetics are typically older (over 40), obese, and initially can be treated with diet alone or diet and oral medications. Diet still is the most important treatment for all types of diabetes. SUGAR BUSTERS! describes a way of eating that is particularly effective for all types of diabetics.

We knew that the way of eating described in this book had to be helpful for diabetics. The response from those who have followed the SUGAR BUSTERS! lifestyle has exceeded our expectations. Many borderline Type II diabetics have seen their blood glucose (sugars) drop back to within the normal glucose range of 90 to 110 milligrams per deciliter. We have seen some Type II, insulin-requiring, diabetics improve to a point where injections are no longer required.

The following is an example that typifies what this way of eating can do for a borderline diabetic. Joe Canizaro, an entrepreneur and prominent

New Orleans developer, recently related his experience with SUGAR BUSTERS! Joe said, "I had my annual physical last week and upon completion of all the usual tests, my doctor said, 'Joe, what in the heck have you been doing?' 'I don't know, Doc, what's wrong with me?' The doctor said, 'Nothing! I have been telling you for six years that you are a borderline diabetic, but this time your blood sugar is normal.'" Joe said, "Well, Doctor, I am on a new way of eating I read about in a book called SUGAR BUSTERS!"

A good example of success by a Type II diabetic who required oral medication for his diabetes is Dr. John Crisp, dean of the College of Engineering at the University of New Orleans. Dr. Crisp was given a copy of SUGAR BUSTERS! by the chancellor of the university, Dr. Gregory O'Brien, who was concerned about John's health. After following the way of eating recommended in SUGAR BUSTERS! Dr. Crisp found that he no longer needed *any* pills and that his quality of life had improved dramatically.

Let's now talk about the experience of Jerry Crowder, a retired executive from Houston, Texas. Jerry, 72 years old, was overweight and a full-fledged diabetic. Jerry was given a copy of our manuscript a month before SUGAR BUSTERS! was published because we knew he was diabetic and knew that our way of eating would be beneficial for him. Sixty days later, one of our authors saw Jerry and asked the standard, "How are you doing?" Jerry replied that he had lost 30 pounds, but what he really liked about our "diet" was that he was *off* of insulin! He said he had been injecting 28 units of Humulin N every morning for the last two and a half years, but that he no longer needed it. He said his doctor told him, "Jerry, your blood glucose was 240 when we started you on the insulin injections, but now it is only 128. You are just a borderline diabetic and you no longer need these injections." Jerry told our author that he now can have a glass or two of wine in the evening without excessively elevating his blood sugar.

These are success stories! What does this mean for Jerry and all those like Jerry who are able to achieve similar results? If diabetics (most, if not all, who are insulin resistant) can keep their blood sugars near normal and eat in a way that requires very little insulin secretion, they will beneficially influence the process that causes the deterioration of their vision, kidneys, nerves, and circulatory system. Diabetics can achieve this goal by eating in a way that does not generate the need for large amounts of insulin. This is one of the major messages this book imparts.

Why is this diet so effective for diabetics? Either a diabetic's pancreas does not manufacture the correct amount of insulin or his or her body does not respond to the insulin in an efficient manner. Most often the culprit is insulin resistance. Insulin resistance means that one's body needs more insulin to maintain its blood sugar in a normal range than does the body of a nondiabetic person who has consumed exactly the same meal. Diabetics following the SUGAR BUSTERS! lifestyle will be less likely to be out of control than they would on many other historically recommended diabetic diets.

Diabetics frequently have damaged kidneys, eyes, nerves, and cardiovascular systems. This may result in diminished circulation ultimately causing loss of extremities. Injections of insulin, although designed to control elevated glucose in a Type II diabetic, often are inefficient. Injected insulin is delivered at predetermined rates that often do not exactly coincide with the requirement created by the consumption of differing amounts of various foods. A properly functioning pancreas in a body that utilizes insulin normally will secrete insulin into the bloodstream in precisely the required amounts at exactly the right time. This precision is not yet achievable with devices that "mechanically" deliver insulin. So, a diabetic should not eat in a fashion that creates a big demand for insulin.

The most severe damage often occurs in diabetics whose blood sugar levels remain the most out of balance. A diet low in refined sugar and processed grain products does not cause gross elevation in blood sugars in the first place, so there is not as much exposure to organ damage.

Diabetes is a very common disease. Every year more and more cases of diabetes are diagnosed, and the percentage of the population having diabetes increases (Figure 6, page 81). In 1900 less than 1 percent of the U.S. population had diabetes. By the year 2000 it is estimated that a minimum of 7 percent to 8 percent, or one out of every twelve people living in the United States, will suffer from diabetes. The diabetes epidemic is a world-wide phenomenon. The common usage of refined sugar is a worldwide phenomenon. Over 100 million people in all countries have diabetes, and that number will grow to 250 million by 2015.

The occurrence of diabetes increases with age for all groups and also with obesity (Figure 7, page 82). The Pima Indians in the southwestern United States have the highest incidence of diabetes in the world (Knowles et al., 1990). As mentioned in Chapter XI, when large-kernel hybridized corn was substituted for the traditional small-kernel, fibrous ears of corn, the rate of diabetes among the Pimas soared to 50 percent! The glycemic indexes of many of the Pima Indians' traditional foods were low compared to the hybridized, highly refined carbohydrates, and their systems could not efficiently handle the increased sugar load (Miller, 1996).

A strong word of caution: If you are currently taking insulin or other diabetic medication and start the SUGAR BUSTERS! way of eating, consult your doctor because you will probably not require your current dose of medication. It is very

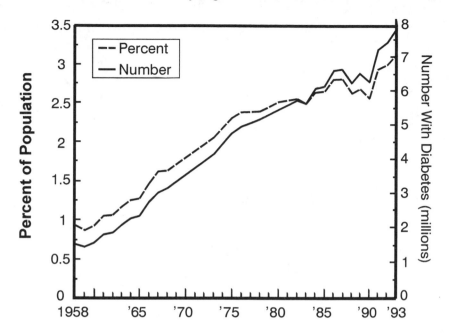

Figure 6.

Increasing incidence of diagnosed diabetes in the United States

Source: Reprinted with permission from Diabetes 1996: Vital Statistics, 1996 American Diabetes Association, Inc.

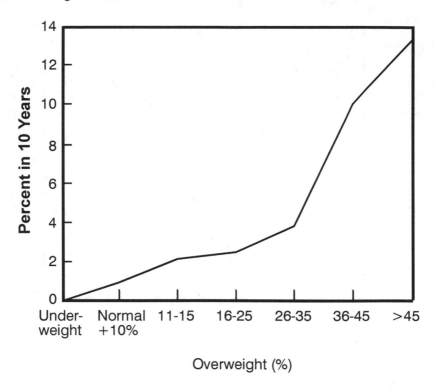

Figure 7.

Likelihood of developing diabetes within 10 years related to percent overweight at initial examination

Source: Reprinted with permission from Diabetes 1996: Vital Statistics, 1996 American Diabetes Association, Inc.

likely that you will not need as much insulin and quite possibly, if you are a Type II diabetic, none at all if you closely follow this diet.

What about Type I (juvenile) diabetics, whose bodies do not manufacture much insulin? Does this diet work for them? Yes, it does! By not eating meals rich in refined or processed carbohydrates (sugar) which create a large requirement for insulin, then Type I diabetics will not need as much additional insulin to keep their blood glucose in a normal range. A Type I diabetic will always require some dose of insulin; however, as stated, eating in this fashion promotes lower mean insulin requirements and is certainly healthier. Remember, our bodies did not evolve on diets that created a great need for high insulin levels.

We previously mentioned gestational diabetes. Although gestational diabetes is temporary, it does indicate a tendency for the mother to be susceptible to Type II diabetes. Over time, 50 percent to 70 percent of gestational diabetics develop Type II diabetes. Those who are obese before or after pregnancy develop it at higher rates. Importantly, untreated gestational diabetes can have a major impact on both the mother and the unborn child. All pregnant women should be screened for gestational diabetes between the twenty-fourth and twenty-eighth week of pregnancy.

As illustrated, just fifteen hundred years ago refined sugar did not exist and neither did the hybridized, plump, and juicy vegetables and grain products that have a much lower fiber content and a much higher glycemic index. Highly processed flours and grains, such as today's white rice, did not exist because the technology was not available to accomplish such complete refining and fiber removal. According to the U.S. Department of Agriculture statistics (Figure 2, page 19), Americans are consuming an average of approximately 150 pounds per person per year of refined sugar (that is over one third of a pound per person per day!). Add to that the consumption of large amounts of plump, low-fiber, and high-glycemic carbohydrates we eat, and we have individuals with a glucose overdose for their underdesigned digestive systems.

Does sugar (carbohydrate) consumption cause or aggravate diabetes? It certainly does aggravate diabetes, and recent statistics strongly suggest that excess sugar consumption is either directly or indirectly causing diabetes or at least speeding the onset of diabetes by causing so many people to become obese and/or insulin resistant. Let us examine the statistics. The rate of diabetes in the United States has more than tripled since 1958, which correlates closely with the increased amount of sugar consumption (Figure 2, page 19). What else are we consuming in amounts so different from what our recent forebears ate? Certainly not fat; the percentage of fat consumed per person since the late 1970s has actually *decreased* from 40 percent to 33 percent, and, more important, the actual consumption in grams per person per day is *down* from 85 grams to 73 grams (a 16 percent drop). Yet the incidence of obesity has doubled since the late 1970s and people weigh eleven to twelve pounds more than when they were consuming larger quantities of fat!

Because a greater percentage of obese people develop diabetes and more people are obese today, is it any wonder the rate of diabetes has tripled since 1958? What other product are we consuming at such an increasing rate than sugar? Colas? Coffee? Well, colas have historically contained huge quantities of sugar, so the consumption of the average cola really is just an increased consumption of sugar. Thank goodness many of the colas are now of the diet type and do not contain refined sugars. Do we really think that coffee causes diabetes or obesity? We don't think so. Coffee is not a problem unless you add large amounts of sugar.

Because the rate of obesity in the United States for both children and adults has doubled since the 1960s (with most of the increase since 1980), and because sugar consumption has gone up another 20 percent just since 1980, what better correlation does anyone want between sugar consumption and what is causing us to get fat? Is not the answer to this dramatic increase in the rates of obesity and diabetes so blatantly obvious that it defies logic for everyone not to see it? How much more obvious can the connection between sugar consumption and obesity and diabetes get?

Add to this the fact that the correlation also makes physiological sense. Most people with diabetes were fat before they became diabetic. *Guyton's Medical Textbook of Physiology* (1986), the doctor's "bible" on physiology, indicates that most sugars or carbohydrates are converted to fat when consumed. Some of the glucose is converted to glycogen to be used for immediate energy needs. The body's ability to store or hold glycogen is limited to only a few hundred grams. The glucose that is not readily used or converted to glycogen is converted to fat. The body can store *thousands* of grams of fat (there are 2.2 pounds in each thousand grams or each kilogram). This is not nutritional theory, but physiological fact. It is very easy to see the converted sugar as fat on ourselves or on our friends!

Couple Guyton's facts on physiology with the additional facts from Wilson and Foster's *Textbook of Endocrinology* (1992; see also Figure 1 of this book on page 16) and the answers are very apparent. They are simple, straightforward, and best yet, logical. The answers make good common sense, unlike the claims of most of today's diets. If we would not eat so much refined sugar and high-glycemic carbohydrates, the major portion of our population would not have these problems!

Again, because of their altered insulin requirements, diabetics should not suddenly change to any new diet without professional medical advice. Unfortunately, American medical schools do not include much nutrition and dietetics in the curriculum. Please urge your doctor to read this book, critique it, check its conclusions with factual data in medical textbooks, and see if he or she does not arrive at a similar conclusion as that found in SUGAR BUSTERS!

Because the high mean levels of insulin promote or accelerate obesity, hypertension, and heart disease, ask your doctor why so many nutritional "experts" still are recommending a carbohydrate-rich diet that causes more insulin to be required by our bodies.

The success stories have been exhilarating. There is significant help available for both the borderline and the full-fledged diabetic. We emphatically predict that, as more research is conducted, the general way of eating presented in this book, which is closer to the way our distant ancestors ate, will ultimately replace the current, faddish diets.

VII | Hypoglycemia

Hypoglycemia is a very common problem in our population. The term *hypoglycemia* is used to indicate a low blood sugar level, usually below 50 mg/dL in adults. A blood sugar level below 40 mg/dL often requires medical attention. A person does not have to be a diabetic to suffer from it. Hypoglycemia frequently is the cause of the midday doldrums that many of us have experienced several hours after lunch. In the majority of instances, we have had a sugar-rich or high-glycemic, carbohydrate-rich meal that initially causes our blood sugars to rise with an associated significant insulin spike (Figure 3, page 45). But when the insulin does its work and the blood sugar begins to fall, it often drops to below normal, resulting in a low blood sugar.

The symptoms of hypoglycemia vary between lethargy and anxiety. Our first response often is to want to eat something, usually another high-glycemic carbohydrate that elevates our blood sugar, making us feel temporarily better. As a result, our blood sugars and insulin levels have fluctuated up and down in a definitely unhealthy fashion that could have been avoided by eating properly.

There are three categories of hypoglycemia: (1) iatrogenic, such as conditions surgically induced following procedures involving the gastrointestinal tract; (2) spontaneous, such as conditions caused by tumors of the pancreas; and (3) reactive hypoglycemia, which we have discussed and is by far the most common form. Insulin and oral hypoglycemic agents are the most common medications responsible for hypoglycemia. Persons with significant symptoms of hypoglycemia should certainly consult their physicians for competent professional advice. However, in the majority of cases, hypoglycemia is purely a result of eating a meal rich in high-glycemic carbohydrates. You frequently can avoid the symptoms associated with a low blood sugar level by following the SUGAR BUSTERS! lifestyle. And just think how much better your performance will be at work and even at play.

VIII | Diet and the Cardiovascular System

Most of us follow a specific diet for one or two reasons. These are usually to enhance our appearance or improve our cardiovascular health. From an appearance point of view, being slender seems to be considered more attractive by both men and women in America today. Most of us have tried, successfully or unsuccessfully, to shed a few extra pounds before vacation or some equally important event. More recently, dieting to improve our health has been gaining greater importance. The cardiovascular system often is the end point of these efforts. Therefore, we would like to elaborate a little about the importance of the cardiovascular system and the influence of diet.

Diseases of the cardiovascular system—primarily

heart attack, hypertension, and stroke—are public enemy number one, accounting for twelve million deaths annually. Coronary heart disease is the leading cause of death in industrialized countries, and in the next ten years, coronary artery disease and stroke will be the leading cause of death in most developing countries.

Heart disease, stroke, and, frequently, hypertension are due to the deterioration of arteries through a process called *atherosclerosis, arteriosclerosis,* or just plain hardening of the arteries. This process is a natural phenomenon of aging. As we get older, so do our arteries. The smooth inner lining called the intima begins to crack when the middle elastic, muscular layer can no longer fully recoil after a pulse wave has expanded the vessel. In these cracks, platelets, fibrin, calcium, cholesterol, and fat accumulate, creating an *atheroma,* or *plaque.*

With continued stress on the arterial wall and further intimal (the innermost coat) disruption associated with blood flow turbulence, more material is deposited until the artery is narrowed significantly, producing reduced blood flow to the corresponding area of the body. We now refer to the process as a disease; its presence has caused a problem.

A frequent question asked physicians is, "How do I avoid getting arteriosclerosis?" The answer is easy. Don't live long enough. But most patients do not like this alternative. However, some factors predispose one to premature or early arteriosclerosis and subsequently to cardiovascular disease. It is important to be aware of the risk factors and plan for them accordingly. Some we can alter. Others we cannot. But the knowledge gleaned from being aware of them usually is very helpful in assisting us to enhance cardiovascular fitness or health.

Initially, there were thought to be three major factors influencing early or premature development of arteriosclerosis: (1) elevated cholesterol; (2) elevated blood pressure; and (3) smoking. However, we now know that many more factors significantly influence the process. These include the following: heredity, diabetes, elevated cholesterol, obesity, stress, sugar, and sedentary lifestyle (Figure 8, page 95).

Heredity, of all these factors, is the most important. Genetic factors contribute to an individual's

Figure 8.

Arteriosclerotic cardiovascular disease risk factors.

Heredity	Elevated triglycerides*
Smoking	Obesity*
High blood pressure*	Stress*
Diabetes*	Sugar*
Elevated cholesterol*	Sedentary lifestyle

*Risk factors beneficially affected by the SUGAR BUSTERS! lifestyle.

susceptibility or resistance to cardiovascular disease. In addition, a substantial part of the susceptibility and response to dietary factors is genetic in origin. Absolute control of the hereditary factor would involve picking our own parents, but for most of us this is not an option! Those individuals with a strong family history of arteriosclerotic cardiovascular disease should be especially aware of the other risk factors so they can alter their lifestyles to minimize the negative influence on their systems.

Smoking is a factor we all have the ability to control. The use of tobacco in all forms promotes the development of arteriosclerosis through a variety of mechanisms. The nicotine in tobacco is a powerful constrictor of blood vessels, causing reduced blood flow and a greater workload on the heart. Smokers have lower levels of plasma antioxidants. We believe this makes them more susceptible to early plaque formation in arterial walls. The beneficial effects of many otherwise successful operations for complications of arteriosclerosis, such as coronary artery bypass, are more than cut in half by patients continuing to smoke.

Diabetes mellitus has long been associated

with early, diffuse, and often prematurely fatal arteriosclerosis. However, the diabetics most severely affected are the 85 percent or so who are insulin resistant. These individuals require increasingly higher plasma insulin levels to achieve the same result in regulating blood glucose. Elevated plasma insulin appears to promote fat deposits and smooth-muscle growth in arterial walls. Both of these processes are involved in plaque formation. In addition, high levels of insulin probably produce increased coagulability, which obviously leads to easier clot formation and arterial occlusion.

High blood pressure, or *hypertension*, is classified as "essential" in over 90 percent of instances. This means that we really do not know its cause, but we do know that it produces extra stress on both the heart and the arterial system. The diastolic, or bottom, pressure in the blood pressure reading is the force or resistance the heart and blood vessels are subjected to during the relaxation phase of the cardiac cycle, or heartbeat. The greater the stress during this phase, the more accelerated the aging, or deterioration, of the arterial walls. This leads to loss of elastic tissue, cracking, and, as seen, plaque formation. Certainly, controlling blood pressure reduces stress on the cardiovascular system and promotes better long-term wear.

Hyperlipidemia (increased fat in the blood), especially *hypercholesterolemia* (elevated cholesterol), is associated with early arteriosclerosis. Cholesterol is an important component in the formation of plaque. Cholesterol also is vital to the proper function of many bodily processes, such as steroid formation and the synthesis of lipoproteins (fat and protein combinations present in the blood) that are both necessary for vital metabolic activities. Researchers also believe there is a link between cholesterol and insulin, as insulin-resistant diabetics, those with high plasma levels of insulin, have abnormally elevated cholesterol levels. The predominant cholesterol component in these individuals is the low-density lipoprotein (LDL) fraction, which frequently is referred to as "bad" cholesterol; remember, for LDL, *L* means lethal. Some components of cholesterol, such as the high-density lipoprotein (HDL) fraction, especially HDL-2 and HDL-3, exert a protective effect on the cardiovascular system; remember, for HDL, *H* means healthy.

Gender is a factor in the development of arteriosclerosis, and, in this instance, women have an advantage at least until menopause. As seen in the next chapter, estrogen in premenopausal women decreases blood plasma insulin levels. This imparts a significant protective influence on the cardiovascular system against the development of arteriosclerosis. After menopause the incidence of arteriosclerosis in women begins to approach that seen in men.

Even in the absence of all risk factors, arteriosclerosis will occur; it is the natural aging process of our arteries. The theoretical maximum life expectancy of the cardiovascular system is approximately one hundred and twenty years. There is a fine line between arteriosclerosis as an aging process and as a disease. In the elderly its presence often is termed normal aging, only to be reclassified as a disease when problems related to it arise. Rest assured, if we live long enough, we will develop arteriosclerosis, but consider the alternative!

Obesity has long been associated with early cardiovascular system problems. In age-adjusted populations where obesity is low, life expectancy is greater. Just compare France and the United States. Between the ages of sixteen and fifty, the French have 50 percent less obesity and 20 percent less cardiovascular and cholesterol problems than their U.S. counterparts. Excess body fat is deposited throughout all body tissues, and the cardiovascular system is no exception. The additional weight imposed by the extra pounds also creates an extra workload for the cardiovascular system.

A sedentary lifestyle, or more aptly stated lack of exercise, definitely does not have a positive influence on the cardiovascular system. Inactivity may not be significantly harmful, but reasonable exercise is beneficial. Exercise decreases blood pressure, decreases serum lipoproteins, especially the bad cholesterol components, decreases obesity, decreases insulin resistance by increasing insulin sensitivity, decreases basal insulin levels, stimulates clot resorption, and reduces the tendency for clot formation. However, the most common problem with exercise programs is that most people's intentions exceed their actual performance.

The maximum cardiovascular benefit can be achieved by exercising on a regular basis, four times a week, so that you elevate your resting heart rate to a prescribed level for a period of twenty consecutive minutes. To determine your ideal heart rate during exercise, you should subtract your age from 220 and multiply this number by 0.70, or 70 percent. This is the heart rate you should sustain for twenty minutes during an exercise program four times a week. If you choose to exercise more frequently and/or for longer periods of time, that is your prerogative, but from a cardiovascular standpoint, exercising to elevate your heart rate to the prescribed level four times a week achieves the maximum cardiovascular benefit from exercise. As a word of caution: if you are over fifty years of age, have cardiac risk factors, or are not accustomed to exercising, consult your physician before beginning your exercise program.

Exercise is a tremendous adjunct to the SUGAR BUSTERS! lifestyle. Both help us lower our mean insulin levels, and that is the goal we are all trying to achieve for healthier and longer lives. Therefore, exercise positively influences many of the risk factors governing the fitness of our cardiovascular systems.

"We are what we eat" is an old adage familiar to almost everyone, but today this is becoming especially more important as we better understand the full spectrum of nutrition and its effect on our various organ systems, especially the cardiovascular system. What we eat may no longer be as important as what happens to it and what metabolic effects it ultimately imparts.

Although fats and meats, especially red meats, have fallen into disfavor, and carbohydrates are definitely "in," has anyone stopped to think about what happens to excess sugar that is the end product of carbohydrate metabolism? Some sugar is used in our blood to maintain an adequate circulating blood glucose level, and some will replenish glycogen stores in the liver and muscles. But what happens to the rest? It is converted to *fat* (Guyton, 1986). Yes, most of our body fat comes from ingested sugar, not ingested fat. This conversion is facilitated by the hormone insulin.

In addition, insulin tends to block lipolysis, the conversion of fat back to glucose. So, individuals with elevated insulin levels have a more difficult time burning fat for energy. Simply stated, they have a hard time losing weight!

Dietary sugar is now recognized as an independent risk factor for cardiovascular disease. This is caused by sugar's effect on insulin secretion. Insulin is now recognized as being atherogenic, that is, it causes the development of arteriosclerotic plaques in or on the walls of blood vessels. In addition, insulin is now known to cause cardiac enlargement, more specifically left ventricular hypertrophy. The left ventricle is the main pumping chamber of the heart and the chamber involved in 99 percent of heart attacks.

Insulin plays a very important role by influencing many of the other factors we have been discussing. An increased insulin level also promotes fat deposition and growth of smooth-muscle cells in the arteries (both necessary to plaque formation) and thus increases the tendency for clot formation. Two factors already discussed, estrogen and exercise, both decrease insulin resistance and are known to have a beneficial effect on the cardiovascular system in retarding the arteriosclerosis process.

However, one group of individuals, regardless of how well they positively influence most of the significant risk factors, appear to develop an early, diffuse type of arteriosclerotic cardiovascular disease that often leads to premature heart attacks, stroke, and complications of hypertension. This group is comprised of insulin-resistant diabetics in whom the only primary measurable abnormality is elevated insulin levels. It has become readily apparent to us, as well as others, that insulin has many influences on the recognized processes responsible for the development of cardiovascular disease through arteriosclerosis. Therefore, the key to improving performance and health through nutrition involves insulin.

Modulating insulin secretion through diet may just be the most important variable influencing the development of cardiovascular disease. Chapter X will discuss how this modulation is accomplished, as well as how it affects weight gain or loss.

IX | Women and Weight Loss

Yes! Many women have more problems losing weight than men. However, some of SUGAR BUSTERS!'s greatest successes have been among women. One lady we know was able to lose 79 pounds over five months on the SUGAR BUSTERS! lifestyle.

Maggy Drezins is a fifty-one-year-old lady from New Orleans who has had a weight problem all of her life, until recently. When she graduated from high school, she weighed 120 pounds, but shortly after marriage and having children, her weight increased to 180 to 190 pounds. Following the sudden death of her husband, she began to eat excessively, finally reaching 319 pounds. Realizing something must be done, she reduced her food consumption and eliminated as much fat as she could from her diet and over eighteen months reduced her weight back to her historical 190 pounds, where she again plateaued. Maggy was introduced to the SUGAR BUSTERS! lifestyle, and over the next five months on SUGAR BUS-TERS! she was able to lose 79 pounds, dropping to her current weight of 111 pounds. She says that SUGAR BUSTERS! is the most fantastic diet ever. She has always been a sweet freak, yet this way of eating has taken away her craving for sweets. Her energy, performance, and sense of well-being are all better. To help keep herself on track, Maggy makes a point of reviewing SUGAR BUSTERS! every month and even refers to the book as "my bible." Following the SUGAR BUSTERS! lifestyle has created a new figure and a new life for Maggy, who has recently married again. Maggy says, "I think SUGAR BUSTERS! is great!"

Another lady, Lala Ball Cooper, from Memphis, Tennessee, wrote the following about her experience with SUGAR BUSTERS!:

My SUGAR BUSTERS! journey began eighteen months ago. How I found the motivation even to begin the trip is still a conundrum. I had, after all, long before that particular spring, completely abandoned any hope of unloading any portion of my substantial cushion of padding that surrounded what really was in fact a medium frame. A literal lifetime of weight battling stretched behind me as far as my memory could track—to early elementary school at least. Forever in search of a solution, and perennially unsuccessful in finding one, I had tried every year's dieting fad one right after the other until I had finally arrived at the point where the news of a possible new solution—even one accompanied by the glitziest media promo—could no longer pique my interest. I can't, then, explain how I found the motivation even to investigate the SUGAR BUSTERS! book. I am still amazed that I bought a copy and even more amazed that I read it and tried it in the first place, so high was the level of skepticism at the time and so low the level of hope that any plan would ever succeed for me.

SUGAR BUSTERS! began to work immediately. Pounds started to fall away swiftly, but I was so heavy when I began that no one noticed at the high school where I teach, even after two months. I told no one that I was dieting (we perpetually fat folks finally learn not to advertise after so many failures). With my secret still intact, I spent the summer continuing to lose steadily. After I returned to teaching in the fall with a noticeably smaller body, my secret was out.

I am now 124 pounds lighter than when I began. Although I lost the bulk of my weight during the first eight months, I still continue to lose, although much more slowly now. The best part of all is that I haven't gained any weight back. To accomplish this I've approached my new success with a new attitude. I know that SUGAR BUSTERS! for me is not something that I will have the luxury of discarding after I reach my desirable weight. It is going to have to remain a habit of life if I intend to keep my weight off. Because it is based on valid nutritional principles and has eliminated the big enemy of dieters, deprivation, continuing this plan is something that I feel that I can reasonably expect to do over the long haul. I am healthier than I have ever been, as attested to by the blood chemistry reports I get from my doctor when I go for annual checkups. For the first time ever I really believe that I am going to be able to put a heavy-weight history behind me.

Congratulations Lala Ball Cooper!

However, some women on SUGAR BUSTERS! have become frustrated because of experiencing slower results in weight loss than their male counterparts. Michel Montignac's most recent book, *La Méthode Montignac Spéciale Femme*, addresses this problem.

Montignac identifies four points that he feels make it more difficult for women to lose weight. These are: (1) women are more sedentary than men; (2) women snack more than men; (3) women diet more than men, so their bodies are more resistant to diets; and (4) women frequently are on hormone supplementation, which makes it more difficult to lose weight and actually may cause them to gain weight. Although the authors of SUGAR BUSTERS! are not in total agreement with Montignac, we do feel there is merit to some of his points.

In general, women may exercise less vigorously and have less muscle mass to burn energy sources than their male counterparts do. More men jog or use highly resistant exercise machines, while women tend to participate more in aerobic exercise programs. However, you must remember that thousands of people are losing weight by closely following the SUGAR BUSTERS! way of eating even in the absence of exercise.

Women who do not work tend to snack more than either working women or their male counterparts. This is only natural because someone frequently in and out of the kitchen has more opportunity to eat than someone who is away from home most of the day.

Women taking certain hormone supplements, such as birth control pills, can have significant problems in losing weight, especially if progesterone is involved. Progesterone increases appetite and definitely promotes fat storage. Many gynecologists use progesterone as an appetite stimulus in patients recovering from surgery or other procedures where improved nutrition and weight gain are desirable. If a woman is on hormonal supplementation, she should not discontinue it on her own but should seek medical consultation. If possible, though, with her doctor's assistance, she should either discontinue any progesterone or change the dosage and schedule of administration so that only the minimal amount necessary is taken. Estrogen, however, may be very beneficial to women trying to lose weight because it increases insulin sensitivity. Estrogen, therefore, acts similarly to exercise as an adjunct to the SUGAR BUSTERS! lifestyle. All three assist you in going through the day with lower insulin levels.

Moreover, women are genetically more efficient at fat storage than men. Historically, because of their ability to bear children, women often are required to support two people rather than one. Therefore, their systems are more efficient at storing reserves that are available to support them during and after pregnancy.

The problem many women have in losing weight is real, and they need to review carefully all of the just-listed points in trying to achieve the best results from the SUGAR BUSTERS! lifestyle. Obviously, some factors, such as hormones, are a stronger influence than others. However, for many women, it is important not to dismiss any of the reviewed points. For them, strict attention to every detail will ultimately yield the pleasing and satisfactory results that we are continuing to see in most women on the SUGAR BUSTERS! lifestyle. Finally, many women on the SUGAR BUSTERS! lifestyle have commented that, in spite of achieving only minimal success in losing weight, their dress size has decreased significantly, indicating that a redistribution of weight is occurring. This has led to a greater sense of well-being and improved self-image. Being slim is a fantastic feeling. Do not deny yourself this attainable pleasure!

X | The Diet Concept

Modulating insulin secretion is the key to our SUGAR BUSTERS! diet. Successfully controlling insulin will allow you to unlock improved performance and health through nutrition. To control insulin you must control the intake of sugar, both the refined variety and the kind so abundant and stimulative in many carbohydrates. This is successfully achieved by selecting a nutritional or dietary concept that modulates insulin secretion in a positive fashion.

We cannot survive without insulin, but we can survive a lot better without too much insulin. Therefore, we recommend selecting foods in forms that stimulate insulin secretion in a more deliberate, controlled manner rather than those that cause the immediate outpouring of this hormone.

Eating in this way will result in lower average insulin levels in our blood throughout any given period. This in turn has a markedly beneficial effect on reducing fat synthesis and storage, as well as other influences we have seen insulin have on the cardiovascular system.

Because insulin is the key to our concept, carbohydrates become the cornerstone. The basic building block of all carbohydrates is sugar. Sugar absorbed from our digestive tract into our blood then stimulates insulin secretion to assist in the transport of sugar into cells as an energy source. The type of the ingested carbohydrate ultimately affects the rate of sugar absorption and, therefore, insulin secretion.

Refined sugar and processed grain products, stripped of their coatings or husks, are almost immediately absorbed in a very concentrated fashion, resulting in rapid secretion of large quantities of insulin. This is the case with most candies, cookies, cakes, pies, and pastries. A diet of refined sugar and processed grain products, therefore, produces a rather marked elevation in average insulin levels throughout a twenty-four-hour period. The additional insulin is then available to promote fat deposition as well as many other previously discussed undesirable effects.

However, carbohydrates in an unrefined form, such as fruits, green vegetables, dried beans, and whole grains, require further digestive alteration before absorption. This in turn causes a proportionate reduction in the rate and quantity of insulin secretion—a modulation of insulin secretion. The end result is lower average insulin levels and less fat synthesis, storage, and weight gain. The positive effects on our appearance and cardiovascular system become apparent.

Obviously, not all carbohydrates are bad, but some carbohydrates, refined or pure, are not healthy for many of us. Many diets advocate eliminating almost all fat and meat, especially red meat, from our nutritional intake. Although many people do eat too much fat, some fat is necessary in our diet to synthesize steroids, lipoproteins, and other substances necessary for the proper metabolic operations of our bodies. But again, remember, it is not so much the ingested fat that makes you obese as the ingested carbohydrates that are converted through the influence of insulin to fat.

Likewise, lean meats are important to our nutritional well-being. Not only do they supply much-needed protein, the building blocks of our bodies, but also ingested protein stimulates glucagon secretion. Glucagon, also from the pancreas, promotes the breakdown of stored fat, creating a "fat loss" for our bodies.

The picture should now become clear. A diet concept based on low-glycemic carbohydrates (high-fiber vegetables, fruits, and whole grains with their fiber), lean meats, and fats in moderation biochemically modulates the insulin–glucagon relationship. This will result in overall body fat loss and a reduction of the adverse effects of insulin on our cardiovascular system.

Alcohol in reasonable amounts may be beneficial. Alcohol increases the HDL, or good cholesterol component (both HDL-2 and HDL-3), decreases plasma fibrinogen, and decreases platelet stickiness and aggregation. These actions all tend to reduce the development of arteriosclerosis and are derived from all forms of alcohol. However, red wine appears to be more beneficial than other forms of alcohol.

Grape skins, which are involved in processing red wines, contain a variety of bioflavonoids called vitamin P that further decrease platelet adhesiveness and also interfere with the oxygenation of LDL cholesterol. It is the oxidized form of LDL cholesterol that is detrimental to our cardiovascular systems.

The curve for the relationship between alcohol consumption and mortality is U-shaped and is shown in Figure 9 (page 119). In moderation there is a potential benefit to our cardiovascular system, but in excess the curve changes quickly to the detriment of the consumer. Therefore, responsible use of alcohol is a must.

Contrary to public opinion, alcohol is responsible for considerably more health-related problems than even tobacco. An aspirin a day, coupled with eating red or green grapes, can more safely impart to our bodies all the beneficial effects ascribed to alcohol consumption.

You have now completed the more technical portion of our book, and although we cannot award you with an M.D. in digestion, metabolism, or cardiology, you should be much better equipped to understand the more practical suggestions on eating for good health and weight loss that follow. The conversations with your own doctors and nutritionists or dietitians also should become more interesting!

In summary, the basis of our concept is to have a positive influence on insulin and glucagon secretion through nutrition. This is achieved by eating a diet composed of natural unrefined sugars, whole unprocessed grains, vegetables, fruits, lean meats, fiber, and alcohol (in moderation). Eating these foods in proper combinations also is very important and is discussed in Chapter XII.

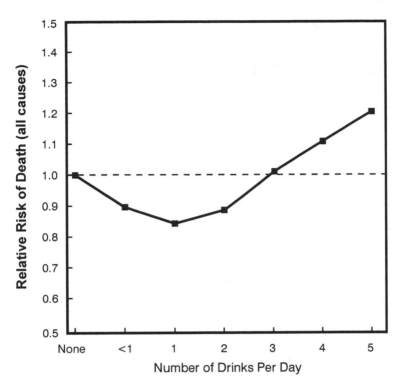

Figure 9.

Deaths from cancer, heart disease, strokes, and accidents.

Source: Modified from Marmot and Brunner (1991).

XI | Acceptable Foods and Substitutes

What foods can we really eat? Principles of metabolism and concepts of nutrition provide us with justification and guidance, but the bottom line of any diet is to choose the proper things to eat. In this chapter we hope to give you the advice and examples to make these choices easy. In addition, we will briefly comment on caffeine, artificial sweeteners, and the spices that are part of our everyday diet.

But first, let's look at some notable exceptions that probably will surprise you. "Potatoes are for pigs and corn is for cattle"—so say the French and with good reason. They fatten these animals just as they fatten us. Potatoes, beets, carrots, and many other root vegetables are simply starch, a storage form of glucose. Once inside our digestive tracts, they are quickly converted to pure sugar. Their absorption is rapid, and the resulting insulin response is very significant.

How many of us, for the sake of dieting, have not eaten a tender, juicy steak but instead have eaten a baked potato with all the fixings? If we scooped out a baked potato and filled the skin with sugar, would you eat it? Certainly not! However, that is exactly what you are doing when you eat a baked potato because it is quickly converted to sugar in your stomach.

Hybrid corn that has large, fleshy kernels causes the same large and rapid insulin response. Maize, the original Indian corn, has smaller kernels and more fiber, therefore has a much more moderate absorption and insulin release. Many of the native American Indians became overtly diabetic when they altered their diets and started eating the modern hybrid variety of corn (Knowles et al., 1990). This again was the result of more than the accustomed sugar load with its expected elevated insulin response.

So, to the list of refined sugar and processed grain products, especially white bread and white rice, now add potatoes, beets, carrots, and corn.

However, the list of recommended foods is quite extensive. Let's see what we *can* eat and enjoy (Figure 10, pages 123–126), as well as what we should avoid (Figure 11, pages 127–128).

In stores in America it is extremely difficult to find many of these meats, vegetables, or cereals (packaged or canned) without one or more of the sugar additives. Also, beware of sauces, such as catsups and most barbecue sauces, that are laced with one or more of the sugars. Most commercial salad dressings contain one or more forms of sugar.

Last, although the glycemic indexes of the listed carbohydrates are moderate to low, you cannot expect to eat three or four portions of beans, sweet potatoes, and so on at a meal and not gain or retain weight!

Figure 10.
Acceptable Foods.

Meats

Lean beef*	Chicken*	Pheasant
Lamb*	Turkey*	Partridge
Pork*	Quail	Elk
Veal*	Venison	Dove
Antelope	Fish	Duck*
Rabbit	Shellfish	
Goose*		
Alligator		

Vegetables

Beans	Squash
Lentils	Zucchini
Peas	Mushrooms
Spinach	Asparagus
Turnip greens	Artichokes
Lettuce	Hearts of palm
Watercress	Okra

Cabbage

Cauliflower

Celery

Broccoli

Cucumbers

Brussels sprouts

Dill pickles

Eggplant

Radishes

Mirliton

Bell peppers

Onions

Sweet potatoes

Fruit

Apples

Tangerines

Lemons

Oranges

Satsumas

Limes

Pears

Mangos

Cherries

Peaches

Berries

Dates

Kiwis

Honeydews

Apricots

Grapes

Grapefruits

Plums

Cantaloupes

Avocados

Tomatoes

Pumpkin

Dairy Products

Milk   Yogurt
Cheese   Cream
Eggs   Butter

Grains and Cereals

Whole-grain products (without dextrose, maltose,
    honey, molasses, brown sugar, or corn syrup)
Whole-grain breads
Whole-grain pasta
Whole-grain brown rice
Wheat bran
Oat bran
Natural grains
Oatmeal

Miscellaneous

Nuts
Spices[†]
Garlic
Chocolate (60% or greater cocoa)

Tabasco sauce

Coffee[‡]

Tea[‡]

Colas with artificial sweeteners[§]

Fruit juices without added sugar (alone)

Olive oil, canola oil

Peanut butter without added sugar

Pure fruit jelly without added sugar

Notes:

[*] Trimmed or skinned.

[†] Spices are generally allowable but have little, if any, nutritional value.

[‡] Most individuals should consume no more than two to three caffeinated beverages daily. Caffeine will potentiate cardiac irregularity, high blood pressure, gastric acid secretion, and appetite. However, sudden cessation of caffeine may produce temporary withdrawal symptoms, such as headache and irritability.

[§] Artificial sweeteners are not harmful to the vast majority of individuals. However, they have no nutritional value.

Figure 11.
Foods to avoid.

Foods to Avoid	Acceptable Substitutes
Potatoes (red or white)	Broiled tomatoes with cheese, sweet potatoes (yams), mushrooms, lentils, or beans
White rice	Whole-grain rice or brown rice
Corn (including popcorn,cornbread, and corn meal)	Okra, peas, asparagus, or squash
Carrots	Broccoli or celery
Beets	Hearts of palm or artichokes
White bread	Whole-grain (stone-ground) breads without added sugars, and whole-grain pasta

Foods to Avoid	**Acceptable Substitutes**
All refined sugar	Nutrasweet or other artificial sweeteners, fructose
Other refined white products, such as cookies, cakes, and so on	Sugar-free ice cream, sugar-free yogurt, sugar-free vanilla ice cream and diet root beer (float)— occasionally

Having learned to make the right choices in each major food group, now we need to look at proper eating patterns and food combinations.

XII | Eating Patterns

All successful nutritional concepts involve the "what," "why," "when," and "how." In the preceding chapters we have discussed the "what" (low sugar) and "why" (regulate insulin secretion), but now we need to address the "when" and "how" that will bring everything together into three full meals and an occasional snack. For many of you, success on the SUGAR BUSTERS! lifestyle will require changing your current eating habits!

Multiple meals stimulate less overall insulin secretion than one or two large feedings because the frequent missing of meals will alter the body's response to insulin secretion and increase fat storage. Therefore, we should strive to consume three balanced meals every day.

As discussed in Chapter III on myths, it is not necessary to count calories. In addition, it is not necessary to count sugar grams, fat grams, or protein grams. Trying to do this not only is frustrating but the results are almost always unreliable. Your daily dietary intake should consist of high-fiber carbohydrates, lean and trimmed meats as sources of protein, and primarily unsaturated fats. SUGAR BUSTERS! is very concerned about your eating *too much fat*, especially saturated fats.

Portion size is very important. The portions of food that you select for each meal should fit nicely on the plate. All of us know what a dinner plate looks like. It has a flat bottom and is flanged around the sides. Your meat and vegetables should fit nicely on the bottom of the plate and should not extend on or over the sides. If you place proper servings on the plate, then the need to count grams is not necessary. Remember, once you have served your plate appropriately, do not go back for seconds or thirds. Everyone should understand this concept, and following it will prevent you from overeating at any particular meal by eating too much of an otherwise glycemically acceptable carbohydrate.

In addition, because most cholesterol is manufactured at night when we are sleeping, a large meal of any type should not be eaten just before going to bed. You should try to finish your evening meal by approximately 8:00 P.M. Once dinner is over, the kitchen is closed—no midnight snacks! Following this advice also should reduce or even eliminate most of the indigestion or heartburn that often awakens us in the middle of the night.

Appropriate snacks are encouraged, and most fruits, except watermelons, pineapples, raisins, and bananas, which have a high glycemic index, are ideal for this occasion. Some individuals who experience frequent indigestion may benefit from eating fruit thirty minutes before or two hours after a meal. Fruit is digested primarily in the small intestine, and when eaten with other solids, its emptying from the stomach is delayed. This permits fermentation that produces indigestion (heartburn) and often gas formation (bloating).

Most fruits contain the basic sugar fructose and stimulate approximately one third of the insulin secretion stimulated by glucose. Consequently, fruit alone as a snack is very beneficial but in combination with other carbohydrates loses the advantage of lower insulin secretion that is achieved when eaten by itself. However, fruit juice may be consumed prior to a meal, such as breakfast, because fluid empties more quickly from the stomach than solids, especially if the juice is drunk first.

In general, fluids should be drunk in small quantities during meals. "Washing" food down frequently causes the bypass of proper chewing that is necessary to break food into smaller, more appropriate particles for better digestion. Excess fluid with meals also dilutes the digestive juices, which reduces their ability to thoroughly interact with food not only in the mouth but also in the stomach. This may result in partially digested food entering the small intestine and can cause cramping.

Fluids may be consumed at your leisure between meals. But be careful because most colas and even popular sport drinks are loaded with sugar and some also contain large quantities of caffeine. Overconsumption of regular coffee and tea also can present the problem of too much caffeine. Caffeine makes the stomach produce gastric acid, which stimulates, not suppresses, appetite. Water and decaffeinated drinks, without added sugar, are preferable. You should make a conscientious effort to drink six to eight glasses of water a day. This is beneficial to the proper function of many of your organs, especially the kidneys. Water consumed throughout the day will lessen your desire for food, thereby helping in weight control.

Alcoholic beverages present a slightly different problem. Alcohol consumed with food (full stomach) is absorbed more slowly, which causes less insulin secretion and potentially less intoxicating effects. Therefore, if you choose to consume alcohol, do so on a full stomach and only in reasonable quantities. As a word of caution, mixers for drinks usually contain a lot of sugar, as does beer (maltose), so neither is considered appropriate for a healthy diet. A dry (low-sugar) red wine is the preferred alcoholic beverage.

Some diets have recommended against mixing certain carbohydrates, such as pasta and rice, with protein. These combinations supposedly stimulate the secretion of competing digestive enzymes. We believe the problem is not so much the carbohydrate–protein combination as the type of carbohydrate that is consumed. For example, a meal of meatballs without added sugar and of whole-grain spaghetti is allowed. As the list in the previous chapter indicates, modest quantities of most unrefined or unprocessed carbohydrates are acceptable. Of course, starches in most forms (except sweet potatoes, which contain a considerable amount of fiber) are harmful and should not be eaten alone or in combination with other foods. Sorry, no meat and potatoes, except for sweet potatoes!

Shoppers beware! Even the best intentions can go awry. Producers of foods have made it difficult for us to eat healthily. Most breakfast cereals, although advertised as being "the best product for your health," are laced with either white sugar, brown sugar, molasses, corn syrup, or honey. In fact, it is difficult to purchase a pure natural-grain cereal. They do exist, but to find them you must closely read the fine print on the side of the box. The same problem applies to bottled, canned, or other packaged foods, sauces, and dressings. Almost all of them have significant amounts of added sugar. Of course, fresh vegetables are your healthiest choice, followed by those that are quick-frozen and those canned or bottled without added sugars.

Whole-grain (stone-ground) and not "whole-meal" breads, rolls, muffins, etc., also are available in most large or specialty grocery stores. But you must be careful that our old nemesis, sugar, has not been added in one form or another. When we really begin to look at what we are eating, we quickly realize just how much sugar is present in almost everything we have been eating. To remind you where this has gotten us, refer to Figure 2 (page 19).

As you now begin to select foods and plan your meals and snacks, remember that sugar and high-glycemic carbohydrates are what you need to watch. Sugar stimulates insulin secretion, which instructs our bodies' metabolism to create, store, and hold fat. In contrast, protein stimulates glucagon secretion, which does just the opposite of insulin. Glucagon instructs our metabolism to mobilize and convert fat back to glucose, which reduces our fat stores and waistlines.

A diet that reduces insulin secretion while enhancing glucagon secretion is the most beneficial.

This method of eating reduces body fat and cholesterol as well as the many health problems caused by both of them. Therefore, good dietary sources of protein are a must. All lean, trimmed meats, such as beef, fish, and fowl, are recommended. These should be grilled, baked, or broiled since frying often involves saturated fats or a batter of processed grains. Other excellent and healthy protein sources are eggs, cheese, and nuts. Remember, it is not necessarily the fat you eat, but the fat you create from sugar, that is ruining your appearance and health.

You should now be getting hungry for what you really like but previously thought you should not eat. Light the grill, and let's see what's for dinner. Figure 12 (pages 138–139) contains an example of a healthy breakfast, lunch, and dinner. This basic diet, with ample calories and fat (but low sugar and low-glycemic carbohydrates) has allowed most of our readers to lose weight, keep it off, and also lower their cholesterol by an average of 15 percent—all this while feeling and functioning better in the process.

Figure 13 (pages 140–141) gives an example of what most of us historically consume in a typical day. The diet in Figure 13, although not necessarily high calorie or high fat, will not let you lose weight, much less cause you to lose weight unless you are blessed with a better-than-average metabolism. The person who consumes a high-glycemic diet consisting of a sandwich with white bread, refined sugar, potatoes, and cookies has a high level of insulin in his body all day and half the night! Why are Americans, the British, and several other westernized countries' populations so obese and fraught with a high incidence of diabetes? Right on! Diets of excessive sugar and high-glycemic carbohydrates "spike" the insulin. *You choose which diet makes the most sense!* Chapter XIV outlines a fourteen-day meal plan, and Chapter XV contains numerous recipes to help you on your way to a successful SUGAR BUSTERS! lifestyle.

Figure 12.

SUGAR BUSTERS! Diet
(balanced toward slimness and health).

Breakfast. Grapefruit, orange, or apple—1/2 hour before; whole wheat and bran shredded wheat, skim milk, and Equal. Or orange juice—1/2 hour before; two eggs cooked in butter; Canadian bacon or pure sausage; a slice of whole-grain toast (with butter); and decaf coffee or tea.

Mid-morning snack. Fruit or almonds, walnuts, or pecans; or peanut butter with whole-fruit jelly (both without added sugar) on rye crackers; or decaf diet drink or coffee.

Lunch. Green salad with olive oil and red wine vinegar or balsamic vinegar, or a sugarless dressing (even blue cheese!); full-size portion of grilled fish or chicken with green or yellow vegetables; whole-wheat matzos or rye crisp crackers; decaf coffee, tea, or water. No dessert.

Mid-afternoon snack. Fruit or nuts or a piece of a high-cocoa-content chocolate (greater than 60% cocoa), or decaf coffee or diet cola or water.

Dinner. Large green salad, steak, lamb chops, veal chops, or hamburger steak; green or yellow vegetables, beans (not canned beans); sautéed (in olive oil) onions, mushrooms, and bell peppers; water or a glass of wine.

Dessert. Sugar-free ice cream and diet root beer (float), or a slice or two of cheese, or a dozen nuts.

Figure 13.

Example of the typical "balanced American diet" (Balanced toward fatness and disease!).

Breakfast. Orange juice with sweet rolls, granola, or cereal (all laced with sugar); biscuits or toast with jelly . . . all bad, except the juice, which, when consumed with sugared or refined carbohydrates, also is bad. Caffeinated coffee or tea, which, although not really bad in moderation, will stimulate some additional gastric acid secretion and can increase your appetite.

Mid-morning snack. More coffee or tea (caffeinated) or a sugar-saturated cola (commonly containing about an inch of liquid sugar).

Lunch. Turkey with mayonnaise on white bread (high-glycemic bread plus fat and sugar in the mayonnaise) or a luncheon salad with a dressing laced with sugar. Caffeinated tea or cola.

Mid-afternoon. Candy and more coffee, tea, or colas.

Dinner. Broiled, skinned chicken (OK), baked potato (ugh!) with margarine, one green vegetable (yea!), rolls (hello, insulin!), fruit salad (so much for rapid stomach emptying), more iced tea or decaffeinated coffee (yea!), and probably a dessert (well, at least it tasted good!).

Before bed. Skim milk and cookies!

XIII | Conclusion

The SUGAR BUSTERS! lifestyle is not another high-fat, low-carbohydrate fad diet. The SUGAR BUSTERS! lifestyle is a nutritional lifestyle. It is logical, practical, and reasonable and involves making healthy and nutritious choices about the foods we eat. The SUGAR BUSTERS! lifestyle supports removing unnecessary fat, especially saturated fat, from our diet. However, we also support eating moderate amounts of lean and trim meats, even red meats, which are healthy sources of protein. Because we recommend avoiding refined sugar and processed grain products that have been added to many foods, most of you will eat fewer carbohydrates than you are currently consuming. More important, success on the SUGAR BUSTERS! lifestyle is a commitment to *choosing correct carbohydrates*. Is this a change in our present nutritional thinking and way of eating?

In health care, transportation, telecommunications, and other fields, tremendous strides have been and are continuing to be made. This is not so for nutrition and dieting. Our ancestors ate better, often out of necessity, than we do today. How they ate is why our digestive system has evolved to what it is today. Sure, vitamins and other food supplements have improved, and we constantly get to eat a variety of foods with their varying vitamins and minerals. But eating in general has caused our health to deteriorate markedly and has prevented a significant increase in life expectancy for middle-aged people. Refining and processing most of what we eat has been an unfortunate nutritional disservice, particularly the introduction of refined sugar. Our health has suffered as a result.

The evidence for this deterioration has been rather obvious for decades. Insulin-dependent diabetics gain weight and their cholesterol continues to rise no matter how carefully they follow their doctor's instructions. Many individuals have given up meat entirely only to have their cholesterol levels increase and their vascular disease progress rapidly.

Nutritionists and dietitians "looked, but did not see." Dufty and Montignac began to see. However, because they were not professionally trained in nutrition, many so-called professionals scoffed at or ridiculed them and even suggested they were charlatans.

The world of nutrition is not flat but round! Previous concepts appeared plausible, but now we have the scientific basis to prove them wrong. Most of our body fat is from ingested sugar (carbohydrates), not ingested fat. This is driven by the effects of insulin and aptly proved in the insulin-resistant diabetic. By modulating insulin secretion through diet, individuals are able to significantly influence body fat, cholesterol, diabetes, and the progression of arteriosclerosis and its subsequent complications. In addition, diet can regulate glucagon secretion, which has additional beneficial effects on fat metabolism.

Eating should be an enjoyable and pleasurable experience and contribute to our performance and health. Many have written about sugar and its harmful effects. We have taken this premise, verified it by current and historical data, and expanded it to include our belief that *insulin* is the key. The nutritional and dietary concepts presented in SUGAR BUSTERS! are consistent with stimulating the ideal levels of insulin and glucagon secretions.

In addition to pleasuring our palates, the concepts proposed in SUGAR BUSTERS! should be good news for the cattle ranchers, sheep ranchers, hog farmers, dairy farmers, and egg producers who recently have been much maligned by various health and nutrition groups. These foods are good for us today just as they were good for our distant ancestors.

With our approach, many individuals already have experienced anticipated weight loss and reduction in cholesterol (an average of approximately 15 percent), as well as improvement in performance, which is so vital to everyone's success. We feel the same opportunity is available to you by following the recommendations on nutrition and diet we offer in SUGAR BUSTERS!

Bon appétit!

XIV | Fourteen-Day Meal Plan

The suggested Fourteen-Day Meal Plan can be consumed in any day-by-day order you desire. If you find a listed breakfast that you would like to eat nearly every day, other than the eggs and Canadian bacon, that is acceptable. Although some of the cereals are rather high glycemic, breakfast is a good time to get your slug of carbohydrates for the day when they are not accompanied by a significant amount of fat.

If you have a low metabolism and store fat very easily, you may want to skip the pastas and breads altogether and substitute one or more of the lower-glycemic carbohydrates listed on Figure 4 (pages 61–65). The best way to consume the fruit juices is to drink them twenty or thirty minutes before the meal, as explained in earlier chapters.

Day 1

Breakfast: Orange juice or grapefruit juice
1 package Quaker instant oatmeal
(regular flavor) made with ⅔ cup
skim, 1% or 2% low-fat milk (microwave on high 2 minutes and 25 seconds;
stir; if desired, sprinkle with Equal)
Coffee, decaf coffee, or hot tea

Lunch: Turkey on whole-grain bread (whole-
grain whole wheat, whole-grain
multi-grain, whole-grain rye or
whole-grain pumpernickel) with
mustard and/or thinly spread lite
mayonnaise, lettuce or fresh spinach,
and tomato
Diet drink, tea, or water

Snack: Apple

Dinner: Pork tenderloin grilled, or baked with
sliced onions
Brown rice cooked with one (14½ oz.)
can of Swansons 100% fat-free and ⅓
less sodium chicken broth and ½ cup
water
Steamed fresh green beans
Water or other appropriate beverage

Dessert: One dozen nuts

Day 2

Breakfast: Orange juice
General Mills Whole Grain Oat
Cheerios and Nabisco/Post Shredded
Wheat 'N Bran tossed together, with
fresh strawberries
Skim, 1% or 2% low-fat milk; if
desired, sprinkle with Equal
Coffee or tea

Lunch: Ham and Swiss cheese on whole-
grain bread with mustard
and/or thinly spread lite
mayonnaise, lettuce, and
tomato
Diet drink, tea, or water

Snack: Thin slice of pâté on 3 Nabisco
Reduced Fat Triscuits or Finn Crisps

Dinner: Salmon, grilled, broiled, poached, or
steamed in microwave with lemon
juice and dill
Broiled or microwaved fresh tomato
half sprinkled with chopped basil
Steamed fresh asparagus

Fresh spinach salad with sliced
mushrooms, olive oil, and vinegar
Water or other appropriate beverage

Day 3

Breakfast:	¹/₂ grapefruit or an orange Uncle Sam Cereal with fresh strawberries or blueberries and milk Coffee or tea
Lunch:	Tuna fish (canned in spring water) with chopped celery and with or without a chopped hard-boiled egg tossed with a little lite mayonnaise on a bed of lettuce Diet drink, tea, or water
Snack:	Low-fat cottage cheese and a fresh peach
Dinner:	Grilled veal chop Fresh mushrooms sautéed in olive oil Whole-wheat pasta (suggest Bionatural Organic Pasta, whole- wheat semolina, or Hodgson Mills whole-wheat pasta) sprinkled with Romano or Parmesan cheese Cooked frozen tiny green peas Water or other appropriate beverage
Dessert:	One dozen almonds

Day 4

Breakfast:	Orange juice or grapefruit juice
	Hot oatmeal
	Coffee/tea
Lunch:	Lean roast beef on whole-grain bread with mustard and/or thinly spread lite mayonnaise, and lettuce, dill pickles, or olives
	Diet drink, tea, or water
Snack:	One dozen grapes
Dinner:	Grilled chicken, or baked chicken rubbed lightly with olive oil and cooked with sliced onion, celery chunks, and sprinkled with salt, pepper, and thyme and/or rosemary
	Grilled sweet potato slices brushed lightly with olive oil, or baked sweet potato
	Cooked frozen baby lima beans
	Water or other appropriate beverage

Day 5

Breakfast:	Orange juice or grapefruit juice
	Puffed Kashi cereal (seven whole grains and sesame, the ready-to-eat cereal or snack) or Kashi the Breakfast Pilaf, with fresh blueberries and milk
	Coffee or tea
Lunch:	Turkey on whole-grain rye or pumpernickel bread with mustard and/or thinly spread lite mayonnaise, lettuce, tomato, and celery sticks
	Diet drink, tea, or water
Snack:	Thin slice of pâté on 3 whole-wheat Triscuits or Finn Crisps
Dinner:	Grilled New York strip or lean sirloin steak
	Fresh mushrooms sautéed in olive oil
	Cooked fresh or frozen spinach
	A sliced ripe tomato with thin slices of fresh mozzarella cheese with dressing of olive oil, balsamic vinegar, a little chopped garlic and

basil with a dash of creole mustard
Water or other appropriate
beverage

Day 6

Breakfast: ½ grapefruit
Tossed Whole Grain Oat Cheerios
and Shredded Wheat 'N Bran with
fresh blueberries and milk, or 2
medium-size buckwheat pancakes
and Smucker's Simply 100%
Spreadable Fruit
Coffee or tea

Lunch: Grilled hamburger with melted
cheese, lettuce, and tomato on
whole-grain bun with mustard
and/or thinly spread lite mayonnaise
or with one slice whole-grain bread
Diet drink, tea, or water

Snack: Orange

Dinner: Grilled lamb chops or lamb sirloin
steak or ground lamb patty
Grilled fresh eggplant slices brushed
lightly with olive oil
Steamed fresh broccoli
Mixed green salad with tomato
chunks and marinated artichoke
hearts (from a jar) sprinkled with

	crumbled blue cheese and tossed with
	olive oil and vinegar
	Water or other appropriate beverage
Dessert:	SUGAR BUSTERS! Chocolate
	Mousse (Chapter XVI, p. 238)

Day 7

Breakfast:	Orange or grapefruit juice
	2 scrambled, fried, poached, or hard-boiled eggs
	Canadian bacon
	Whole-grain toast
	Coffee or tea
Lunch:	Smucker's Natural Creamy or Crunchy Peanut Butter and Smucker's Simply 100% Fruit (Spreadable Fruit) on whole-grain bread
	Skim, 1% or 2% low-fat milk or diet drink, tea, or water
Snack:	Apple
Dinner:	Grilled tuna (or any other fish)
	Steamed or microwaved chunks of fresh red peppers, yellow peppers, onions, broccoli florets, and garlic
	Fresh spinach salad with hearts of palm tossed with creole salad dressing of olive oil, red wine vinegar, and a dash of creole mustard
	Water or other appropriate beverage

Day 8

Breakfast: Orange or ½ grapefruit

                  Hot oatmeal

                  Coffee or tea

Lunch: Turkey and Swiss cheese on rye, whole-grain, or pumpernickel bread with mustard and/or thinly spread lite mayonnaise, lettuce, and tomato

                  Diet drink, tea, or water

Snack: One dozen grapes

Dinner: Ground beef cooked in no-added-sugar tomato sauce (Colavita sauces)

                  Whole-wheat pasta sprinkled with Romano or Parmesan cheese

                  Steamed fresh yellow or spaghetti squash and/or zucchini

                  Romaine lettuce salad with fresh snow peas, roasted pine nuts, and a dressing of olive oil, balsamic vinegar, a little chopped garlic, basil, and a dash of creole mustard

                  Water or other appropriate beverage

Dessert: No-sugar-added (sugar-free) yogurt ice cream

Day 9

Breakfast: ½ grapefruit
Hot oatmeal or Uncle Sam Cereal
and milk
Coffee or tea

Lunch: Chicken salad with tomato wedges
on lettuce
Three Triscuits or one slice of whole-
grain toast
Diet drink, tea, or water

Snack: A dozen almonds

Dinner: Pork chops sautéed with sliced
onions in a small amount of olive oil
Red kidney beans cooked with ham
chunks, chopped onions, and garlic
Brown rice cooked with chicken
broth
One half steamed fresh artichoke,
served with a dip of melted butter or
a dip of olive oil, garlic salt, and
lemon juice
Water or other appropriate beverage

Day 10

Breakfast: Orange juice
            Tossed Whole Grain Oat Cheerios
            and/or Shredded Wheat 'N Bran with
            fresh strawberries and/or blueberries
            and milk
            Coffee or tea
Lunch: Lean roast beef on whole-grain, rye,
            or pumpernickel bread with mustard
            and/or thinly spread lite mayonnaise,
            lettuce, and tomato
Snack: Kiwi fruit and a half dozen nuts
Dinner: Baked turkey breast rubbed lightly
            with olive oil and cooked with sliced
            onions, celery chunks, salt, pepper,
            and thyme
            Baked sweet potato, steamed fresh
            green beans
            Water or other appropriate beverage
Dessert: Two thin slices of cheese

Day 11

Breakfast: Orange juice or grapefruit juice
             Hot oatmeal
             Coffee or tea
Lunch: Cobb Salad (julienned slices of
             turkey, ham, and Swiss cheese with
             or without a hard-boiled egg), no-
             sugar salad dressing
             Three Triscuits or one slice of
             pumpernickel bread
             Diet drink, tea, or water
Snack: Low-fat cottage cheese and
             strawberries
Dinner: Split pea soup
             Venison or grilled marinated flank
             steak
             Sautéed mushrooms
             Steamed fresh cauliflower
             Tomato half with melted blue cheese
             Water or other appropriate beverage

Day 12

Breakfast: ½ grapefruit
Hot oatmeal
Coffee or tea

Lunch: Tuna fish (canned in spring water)
with chopped celery and with or
without a chopped hard-boiled egg
tossed with a little lite mayonnaise
on whole-grain bread

Snack: Fresh peach

Dinner: Grilled skinless and boneless chicken
breast sprinkled with salt, pepper,
onion powder, and garlic powder
Brown rice cooked with chicken
broth, with chopped ripe tomato
heated and placed on rice
Can of Trappey's Black-Eyed Peas,
with or without jalapeño peppers
Romaine lettuce salad with
marinated artichoke hearts (from a
jar) and a dressing of olive oil, red
wine vinegar, and a dash of Dijon
mustard
Water or other appropriate beverage

Day 13

Breakfast: Orange juice or grapefruit juice
2 scrambled, fried, poached, or hard-boiled eggs
Canadian bacon
Whole-grain toast
Coffee or tea

Lunch: Grilled hamburger and melted cheese with lettuce and tomato
Diet drink, tea, or water

Snack: Apple or ½ cup unsweetened applesauce

Dinner: Grilled shrimp or trout (or any other fish) with lemon
Steamed fresh broccoli
Whole-wheat pasta with sauce of chopped fresh tomato and basil sautéed in olive oil and sprinkled with Romano cheese
Mixed green salad with hearts of palm and roasted pine nuts with creole dressing of olive oil, red wine vinegar, and a dash of creole mustard

	Water or other appropriate beverage
Dessert:	No-added-sugar (or sugar-free) ice cream

Day 14

Breakfast:	Orange juice Puffed Kashi Cereal or Kashi Breakfast Pilaf with fresh strawberries and/or blueberries and milk Coffee or tea
Lunch:	Grilled boneless and skinless chicken breast in Caesar Salad, or on lettuce with tomato Diet drink, tea, or water
Snack:	Pear, or slice of melon
Dinner:	Grilled beef filet Wild rice cooked with chicken broth or brown rice cooked with beef broth and chopped onions Sautéed mushrooms or Portobello mushrooms Steamed fresh asparagus Water or other appropriate beverage

XV | SUGAR BUSTERS! Recipes

By popular demand, let us offer a few recipes created by some of the authors, their wives, or their mothers. From this sampling, you will see that many variations can be adapted quickly. Most will be simple and relatively easy to prepare. A few of our old favorites, although taking a little longer, should be worth the extra effort. In the next chapter you will see a sampling of what many of the best restaurants in New Orleans have to offer followers of the SUGAR BUSTERS! lifestyle.

There are many exotic herbs and spices. There are also many common ones, tried and true, that our palates love to taste. The first part of this section centers around recipes that focus on the more common herbs and spices because they did not get to be so popular by being on the fringe of enjoyable taste. A famous New Orleans chef once said, "I can make an almost infinite variety of great flavors by simply using different amounts of three common peppers: white pepper, black pepper, and red pepper."

We must reiterate one point; just because a recipe is listed here as "legal" does not mean you can eat an unlimited amount of these dishes. A double portion of a "legal" carbohydrate can cause the need for the same amount of insulin as is needed from consumption of a single portion of a high-glycemic carbohydrate.

Appetizers

First, let's simply list appetizers that require only the opening of a package or a can or a little warming—no recipes at all!

Cheese Bites or Wedges

All types, whatever your favorites, in moderation.

Meat Cubes

Lean cuts of bite-size meat cubes, cold, skillet warmed, or sautéed in soy sauce or garlic, butter, and salt. This could come from fresh or leftover roast, steak, lamb, chicken, or game. If it is fresh, it must stay in the skillet long enough to be cooked.

Celery Sticks

Celery filled with pimento cheese spread, Velveeta cheese, or other no-sugar cheese-based spreads.

Sardines

Sardines, preferably in olive oil, with additional salt if necessary and a healthy squeeze of lemon juice.

Herring

Herring in sour cream cut to bite size. (The Omega 3 fats from cold-water fish are good for you.)

For a couple of recipes that do require some preparation, try these:

Sautéed Mushrooms

Carton of mushrooms (white, Portobello,
   Shiitake, etc.)
Olive oil
Parsley flakes
Salt to taste
Balsamic vinegar

Sauté mushrooms in a large skillet with about 1/16 inch olive oil, a heavy sprinkling of parsley flakes, a sprinkling of salt to taste, and one tablespoon of balsamic vinegar containing no more than 1 gram of sugar per serving. This should be done over a low to medium fire. Cook until the mushrooms are tender.

Serves 2–4.

Oysters Tony

3 dozen oysters
1 stick butter
1 bunch green onions, cut in 1/2-inch pieces
8 oz. white mushrooms, cut in half
Garlic salt
1/2 cup vermouth or sherry
Triscuit or Finn Crisp crackers
Tabasco

Drain oysters in a colander. Melt butter in a saucepan, and add green onions plus mushrooms. Sprinkle with garlic salt and sauté until vegetables begin to get soft. Turn up the heat and add oysters. Cook for 5 minutes at a medium boil. Add vermouth or sherry during the last couple of minutes of boiling. Dip out oysters, onions, and mushrooms with a spoon and serve on a Triscuit or Finn Crisp. Be sure to add one or more drops of Tabasco on each bite-size serving, and add more garlic salt if necessary. This can also be served as a main course in a bowl and eaten with a fork and spoon without crackers. But don't forget the Tabasco! The juice left over in the saucepan is a high-quality oyster soup.

Serves 4–6.

Salads

Eat a lot of salads because they are important to the overall digestive system. Our ancestors ate a lot of leafy vegetables when they could find them. Make salads with various lettuces or fresh spinach, or mixed with broccoli, cauliflower, bell peppers, mushrooms, or tomatoes.

If you want a fruit salad or a lettuce and fruit salad, we recommend you make an entire meal of it or eat it as a snack and without a sugar- or honey-sweetened dressing.

Salad Dressings

Salad dressings should contain no sugar or very small amounts of sugar. Although there are many interesting variations on the four types of dressings listed, we will give you exact proportions for each one to get you started in making acceptable salad dressings. You also can find dressings like these in a grocery store, but finding them without added sugar is not always easy.

Basic Olive Oil and Vinegar Dressing

2 tbsp. extra virgin olive oil
1 tbsp. red wine vinegar
1/8 tsp. oregano
Less than 1/8 tsp. salt
Juice from 1/8 lime

Mix and pour.

Italian-Style Vinaigrette

Either mild or strong, depending on the amount of garlic and salt:

2 tbsp. extra virgin olive oil
1 tsp. chopped garlic

1/2 tsp. McCormick's Italian Seasoning
1/2 tsp. fresh lemon juice
1/8 tsp. salt

Mix and pour.

Mustard-Based Dressing

1 cup extra virgin olive oil
1/4 cup red wine vinegar
1 heaping tbsp. creole or Dijon mustard
1/4 minced bell pepper (optional)

Mix and pour.

Blue Cheese Dressing

1/2 cup extra virgin olive oil
1/2 tsp. garlic powder
1/2 tsp. onion powder
1/2 tsp. coarse ground black pepper
1/2 tsp. tarragon

$^{1}/_{2}$ tsp. chervil

$^{1}/_{2}$ tsp. Italian seasonings

3 tbsp. white wine vinegar

$^{1}/_{2}$ cup crumbled blue cheese

Combine all ingredients, except blue cheese, in a jar and shake until well blended. Just before serving add crumbled blue cheese to jar and shake once or twice. Pour over salad and serve immediately.

Soups

Basic Chicken Soup

2 cans chicken broth

1 large can whole or chopped tomatoes

1 can no-sugar-added green beans

$^{1}/_{2}$ stalk chopped celery with leaves

1 large yellow onion, quartered

$^{1}/_{2}$ tsp. black pepper

$^{1}/_{8}$ tsp. white pepper

$^{1}/_{4}$ tsp. basil

Pour all ingredients into a saucepan and set over medium heat. Bring to a boil, then turn to medium low, cover, and cook for 30 minutes. You can add chunks of cooked chicken, beef, or ham to make a heartier soup or a dish sufficient for an entire meal. If you like a spicier soup, substitute (or add) a can of Rotel tomatoes.

To put a little extra flavor in clear broths, add some finely chopped green onions, including the tops, or even small bits of chicken, steak, or other meat. Interestingly enough, the broth and bouillon cubes are made mainly from salt, corn syrup, sugar, and chicken or beef. Homemade broths boiled from chicken, beef, or fish bones are the only ones we have seen without added sugar. Of course, unless you are diabetic, the amount of added sugar in a bouillon cube probably won't hurt you.

Serves 6.

Artichoke Soup

$1/2$ stick butter or margarine
$1/4$ cup olive oil

2 small onions, chopped
5 cloves garlic, chopped
Three 14-oz. cans of artichoke hearts in water
Three 16-oz. cans of chicken broth
1 tbsp. parsley
1/2 tsp. basil
1/2 tsp. oregano
2 tbsp. whole-wheat flour
Grated Parmesan cheese

Melt butter and olive oil together. Sauté onions and garlic. Add artichokes and cook a little. Add chicken broth, parsley, basil, and oregano. Cook 1 hour in covered pot. Mix whole-wheat flour in 1 cup of water and add to pot. Cook 15 minutes more. Sprinkle with Parmesan cheese immediately before serving.

Serves 6–8.

Shrimp and Crab Okra Gumbo

2 lbs. fresh okra
4 tbsp. vegetable oil

2 cups onion, chopped

1 small can tomato paste

2 medium tomatoes, chopped, or 1 can of
chopped tomatoes

1/3 cup shallots, thinly sliced

1 cup green pepper, chopped

2 qts. water

1 tsp. Tabasco sauce

3 tsp. Italian herbs

Juice of one lemon

1 tbsp. Worcestershire sauce

2 tbsp. Kitchen Bouquet browning sauce

3 tsp. garlic, minced

2 lbs. gumbo crabs, halved and cleaned, or 1 lb.
white crabmeat

2 lbs. shrimp, peeled and deveined

1/2 lb. low-fat sausage (optional)

Salt to taste

Black pepper to taste

Wash and drain okra. Cut into 1/2-inch slices. In a heavy skillet, sauté the okra in 2 tbsp. oil over medium heat for about 15 minutes. Set aside. In another skillet, sauté onions in 2 tbsp. oil until soft. Transfer to large gumbo pot. Add tomato paste, stirring until blended. Continue to stir while adding chopped tomatoes, shallots, and green peppers. Slowly add 2 qts. of water to vegetable mixture. Add salt, Tabasco, Italian herbs, lemon juice, Worcestershire sauce, Kitchen Bouquet browning sauce, garlic, black pepper to taste. Bring to slow boil and add crabs and shrimp. Add sausage, if desired. Simmer for approximately 1 hour with the pot loosely covered, stirring occasionally. Eat as is or spoon over a little brown rice.

Serves 8.

Meats

Meats are a basic in the SUGAR BUSTERS! way of eating; not necessarily fat meats, but trimmed, lean meats. To stay slim, however, eating a patty of ground beef or hamburger steak with a salad and a green vegetable is better than eating chicken with a baked potato or fish with corn on the cob and slices or rolls of white bread. The following recipes are generally simple, yet tasty, and should get you started in the meat category.

Cajun Pot Roast

For beef, pork, lamb, venison, duck, dove, quail, or, yes, even a mixture of the above!

Meat of your choice
Wishbone Italian salad dressing
Olive oil
Seasonall
Black pepper
4 oz. water

Marinate your roast or birds in Wishbone Italian salad dressing for 2 hours or even overnight. Use an appropriate-size Ziplock plastic bag to reduce the amount of Wishbone dressing required; about half of a large bottle is usually plenty. Cover the bottom of an iron Dutch oven with about 1/8 inch of olive oil. Turn heat to high and brown meat on all sides. Sprinkle moderately to heavily with Seasonall and black pepper. Add about 4 oz. of water, and if you want a richer gravy, add a portion of the marinade. Cover immediately; turn heat to low so liquid drops to a slow bubbling. Cook large roasts for 3 hours and small roasts or fowl for 2 to 2 1/2 hours. Check occasionally to see whether additional water is needed. This recipe is easy and almost foolproof.

Serves 3 per pound of roast.

Hamburger or Hamburger Steak

As a meat dish and not on a bun.

1 yellow onion, chopped
Parsley flakes
2 lbs. lean hamburger meat
Black pepper to taste
Salt

Knead onion, some parsley flakes, and black pepper into the hamburger meat. Separate into thick patties. Sprinkle patties with salt. Cook over medium to medium-low heat until patties are done to your preference. Serve with sliced tomatoes, cheese, or a green salad.

Serves 6.

Italian Meat Roll

1 cup stone-ground wheat bread crumbs
2 beaten eggs
2 tbsp. fresh parsley, chopped
$1/2$ can V8 or tomato juice
1 tsp. salt
$1/2$ tsp. freshly ground black pepper
2 cloves garlic, minced
$1/2$ tsp. dried oregano
2 lbs. lean ground beef
8 slices baked or boiled ham, sliced thin
8 oz. shredded mozzarella cheese

Preheat oven to 350 degrees. Prepare bread crumbs: Place 4 slices of torn wheat bread in food processor and process on high. Combine bread crumbs, eggs, parsley, tomato juice, salt, black pepper, garlic, and oregano and mix. Add ground beef and mix well. On wax paper, shape and flatten meat mixture into a rectangle. Layer ham slices on top of meat and top with shredded cheese, leaving small border of meat edge. Roll up meat, lifting wax paper, starting from short edge. Mold meat to close ends and seam. Place seam edge down in 9-by-12 baking dish. Bake at 350 degrees for approximately 1 hour, or until done. Cut into 1-inch medallions.

Serves 6.

Texas Steak (sirloin, strip, or filet)

Lowry's Seasoned Salt
Celery or onion salt
Garlic powder
Black pepper
Generous squeeze of fresh lemon juice
Capful of apple cider vinegar
Large, 3½ inch-thick piece of steak (4 to 6 lbs.)
1 stick butter

Mix the first six ingredients and rub into both sides of the steak. Let stand at least 2 hours at room temperature or refrigerate overnight. Cook on outdoor grill, turning once, for approximately 1 hour if the steak is 3 inches thick. The smaller the steak, the less time it takes. Cut it and check. Keep top closed to add a smoked flavor and use mesquite wood or mesquite chips to add still more flavor. While the meat is cooking, melt the butter in a saucepan and add the same ingredients as those rubbed on the steak. Be careful not to add too much of the salts. When meat is done to your taste, slice in ¼-inch strips. Pour saucepan liquid over steak slices and serve immediately. Watch out, Ruth!

Serves 6–8.

Smothered Round Steak (or venison)

2 lbs. round steak or venison backstrap, cut into
　　slices ¼-x-3 inches thick
White pepper
Olive oil
2 medium-size onions, sliced
Water

Sprinkle meat with white pepper. Brown in skillet with a small amount of olive oil. Add onions and enough water to cover the bottom of the skillet (about ¼ inch). Cover and cook on medium or low for about 20 minutes or until tender.

Serves 4.

Simple Grilled or Broiled Chicken

A classic healthy dish such as chicken is a must for any way of eating. Healthiest of all would be skinless chicken.

8 skinless chicken pieces
Salt
Pepper
Olive oil
Rosemary (optional)

Cook chicken pieces in a skillet, on a grill, or under a broiler after rubbing chicken with a small amount of salt and pepper and adding a little olive oil. Another spice that goes well with chicken is rosemary, which can be rubbed on along with the salt and pepper. Serve with any "legal" vegetable and green salad.

Serves 3–4.

Stuffed Bell Peppers

10 medium green bell peppers
1½ cups onion, chopped
2 lbs. ground sirloin beef
2 tbsp. vegetable oil
2 tbsp. parsley, minced
1 tbsp. garlic, finely chopped
1 tsp. thyme
1 tsp. basil
2 tsp. salt
1 tsp. freshly ground black pepper
¼ tsp. cayenne pepper
2 tbsp. Worcestershire sauce
28-oz. can chopped tomatoes
3 cups cooked brown rice
1 cup grated Parmesan cheese

Preheat oven to 350 degrees. Slice off tops of green peppers. Remove seeds and membranes and wash peppers under cold water. Set aside. In a large, heavy skillet, over medium heat, sauté onions and ground beef in oil until brown. Add parsley, garlic, thyme, basil, salt, black pepper, cayenne pepper, and Worcestershire sauce. Cook for about 3 minutes, continuing to stir. Drain the chopped tomatoes and add to the mixture. Cook for 5 minutes, continuing to stir. Add the cooked brown rice and mix well. Cover skillet and cook over low heat for another 5 minutes. Remove skillet from heat and add Parmesan cheese. Stir to blend in cheese. Stuff the peppers with the rice mixture. Place the stuffed peppers in a 9-by-12 Pyrex pan to which 1 inch of hot water has been added. Cover pan with foil and bake 45 minutes or until peppers are soft and tender. Remove foil and allow tops to brown (about 5 to 10 minutes).

Serves 10.

Quick Skillet-Grilled Fish

Redfish, speckled trout, snapper, or any nonoily white fish fillets

Garlic salt
Lemon juice
Olive oil
Parsley flakes

Dry the fillets with a paper towel so the fish will not splatter when put into the hot grease. Sprinkle fillets with garlic salt. Squeeze generous amount of lemon juice on fillets. Cover bottom of skillet with olive oil and turn heat to high. When the oil is hot, add fillets and sprinkle with parsley flakes. Cook about 2 minutes, or longer if fillets are thick. Turn, and add more parsley flakes and more fresh lemon juice. After another 2 minutes, put on plates and eat immediately.

Serves 1 person per 2 small fillets.

Sautéed Shrimp

2 lbs. shrimp, peeled and deveined
1/2 stick butter
Garlic salt

Fresh parsley, chopped
Lemon juice

Peel shrimp and sauté in skillet with butter, garlic salt, and chopped fresh parsley. Cook until done, but not tough. Add a generous squeeze of lemon juice 1 minute prior to removing from fire. Serve immediately, spooning any remaining skillet juice over shrimp.

Serves 2.

Cheese Omelet

Various omelets also make a good main dish. For a cheese omelet, simply beat three eggs and mix with shredded cheddar cheese and a little salt, and cook in a nonstick skillet with ¼-inch slice of butter. For a Spanish-type omelet, first sauté some bell peppers and onions in a little canola or olive oil, then add 2 tbsp. salsa (mild to hot); make sure the salsa is warm before stirring in the eggs. If you are really trying to lose weight, instead of eating this with a slice of "legal" toast, simply add one more egg so you will be satisfied. You could also serve it with a grilled tomato covered with Parmesan cheese and a little salt and pepper.

Serves 1 or 2.

Vegetables

The list of allowed vegetables is very long, as can be seen in Figure 10 (pages 123–126), and the list of forbidden vegetables can be counted on just both hands. Raw vegetables usually are best for you (like our distant forefathers ate them), but most people like vegetables that have been cooked.

Steaming various vegetables like broccoli, green beans, cauliflower, squash, etc., is quick, easy, and inexpensive. Just serve them plain or add your favorite spices or sugar-free salad dressing before serving.

A mixture of vegetables that has been sautéed and reasonably seasoned can be both a tasty and colorful addition to any meal. Peppers, onions, mushrooms, zucchini, garlic, and the like are abundantly available to make this dish. Of course, everyone likes variety in vegetable dishes so a few are listed.

Green Beans

1 lb. green beans, washed and snapped
2 tsp. olive oil
$1/2$ tsp. garlic salt

Put beans in a microwave-safe container and cover with plastic wrap. Microwave for 5 minutes or until just tender. Toss with olive oil and garlic salt.

Serves 4.

Pinto Beans with Salsa

1 lb. dried pintos, washed
3 qts. of water
2 large yellow onions, halved

2 tbsp. bacon drippings or 3 slices of raw bacon
Salt to taste

Bring beans to a low boil in the water for 1 hour. Add onions, bacon, and salt. Cook at low boil, covered, for an additional hour. Add more water if necessary so beans will have plenty of liquid. Taste before cooking is completed to see if additional salt is needed.

Serves 4–6.

Salsa

1 can diced Rotel tomatoes
¼ bunch cilantro leaves, chopped fine
½ medium onion, chopped fine
Juice of ½ lemon
A little additional salt if preferred

Mix all salsa ingredients. Serve beans in a small bowl and add as much salsa as desired.

Squash Casserole

2 lbs. yellow squash
2 medium tomatoes, sliced
Salt and pepper to taste
2 medium onions, sliced
½ cup Parmesan cheese
½ stick margarine

Peel and slice squash into rounds about ½" thick. Place ⅓ of the sliced squash in bottom of baking dish, add ⅓ of the tomatoes, salt, pepper, ⅓ of the onions, and ⅓ of the cheese. Dot with ⅓ of the margarine. Repeat with two additional layers. Cover lightly with foil and bake in preheated 350-degree oven for 30 minutes. Remove foil and continue cooking for 10 minutes.

Serves 4–6.

Spicy Lentils

1 lb. dried lentils
1 qt. water
2 tsp. salt

1 medium onion, chopped
1/4 cup extra virgin olive oil
One 10-oz. can Rotel diced tomatoes and chiles

Rinse and drain lentils in colander. Cover with 1 qt. water, add salt, and simmer in covered pan until tender, about 45 minutes. Check pan frequently and add water if needed. In small skillet, sauté the onion in olive oil until tender. Add onion, olive oil, and drained tomatoes to the lentils, stirring carefully. Cook for 10 to 15 minutes. Add more salt if needed.

Serves 4–6.

Stuffed Eggplant

2 medium eggplants
1 small onion, chopped
2 tbsp. chopped shallots
4 tbsp. margarine
1 lb. medium, peeled, cooked shrimp
1/2 lb. white crabmeat
2 tbsp. parsley
1 beaten egg

Juice of 1 lemon
1 tbsp. Worcestershire sauce
Salt and pepper to taste
1/2 cup grated Parmesan cheese

Cut eggplant in half. Scoop out the pulp and place in enough boiling water to cover. Lower heat and simmer 5 minutes. Drain eggplant and set aside. In medium skillet, sauté onions and shallots in melted margarine until vegetables are soft. Add eggplant, shrimp, crabmeat, parsley, and beaten egg to skillet. Add lemon juice, Worcestershire sauce, and salt and pepper to taste. Spoon mixture into eggplant shells. Sprinkle with Parmesan cheese. Place eggplants in Pyrex dish in which 1 inch of water has been added. Bake in 350-degree oven until brown, approximately 30 minutes.

Serves 4.

Eggplant Parmesan

2 medium eggplants
Vegetable oil

5 cups basic tomato sauce (see following recipe)

½ lb. provolone cheese, sliced thin

⅔ cup Parmesan cheese, grated

Salt and pepper to taste

Peel eggplants and slice into ½-inch ovals. Rinse and drain eggplant slices. Salt and pepper eggplant and set aside. Spray 9-by-12 rectangular glass baking dish with vegetable oil. Cover bottom of dish with about 1½ cups of tomato sauce. Place a layer of sliced eggplant over the sauce. Place single slices of provolone cheese over the eggplant and sprinkle with ½ of the Parmesan cheese. Cover with 1½ cups of tomato sauce. Add remaining eggplant slices, and cover with additional provolone slices and Parmesan cheese. Top with remaining tomato sauce. Cover dish with aluminum foil, and bake at 350 degrees for 30 to 45 minutes, until eggplant is fork-tender. Uncover and continue to bake for 10 to 15 minutes to reduce the amount of liquid.

Serves 6.

Variation. Chicken or Veal Parmesan

Salt and pepper 8 boneless chicken fillets or 8 veal cutlets. Sauté in 2 tablespoons of margarine and 2 tablespoons of olive oil until lightly browned. Drain on paper towels. Substitute chicken or veal fillets for eggplant in recipe.

Basic Tomato Sauce

1 medium onion, chopped
3 cloves garlic, chopped fine
3 tbsp. extra virgin olive oil
One 28-oz. can crushed tomatoes in purée
One 15-oz. can tomato sauce with no added sugar
1/2 cup fresh basil, chopped, or 1 tsp. dried basil
1 tsp. baking soda
Salt and pepper to taste

In a medium skillet, sauté the onion and garlic in the olive oil until tender. Add the crushed tomatoes and tomato sauce, stirring to mix, while cooking over medium heat. Add the basil and baking soda, continuing to stir. Lower heat to a simmer. Add salt and pepper to taste. Simmer for 15 minutes, stirring frequently.

Makes about 5 cups of sauce.

Desserts

This is the most difficult category for anyone trying to lose weight or to stay off sweets to generally improve health. Let us mention a couple of
substitution thoughts. Try eating a few nuts after
a meal (almonds, walnuts, peanuts, pecans, etc.).
For some reason this seems to satisfy the sweet
craving within minutes in most people. One large
spoonful of unsweetened peanut butter also can
do the trick. Just don't place a spoonful of peanut butter in your mouth if you are expecting a
phone call!

Another substitute that also works well when
eating out is to have soup or something else as an
appetizer and save the leafy salad for the dessert.
This is the way the French commonly eat, and
they certainly don't have as many obesity or
cardiovascular problems as most other Western
countries.

Cheese also makes a good dessert. But don't eat
cheese or much of any fat if you happen to have
had a significant amount of carbohydrates (bread,
rice, etc.) during the same meal.

Sugar-free or no-added-sugar ice creams and yogurt, in moderation, won't generally add pounds to most people. However, not all of us have the same metabolism, and these ice creams, although they have not put weight on the authors, may not work for everybody. We have been unable to find glycemic index data on several of the sugar substitute ingredients, such as maltodextrin, sugar alcohol, or sorbitol, in those products. We recommend avoiding foods with large amounts of the sweeteners because they are all carbohydrates and will ultimately be broken down into sugar in our system. If these sweeteners are listed high in the list of ingredients, it probably means that large amounts of them have been used; therefore, these foods should be avoided. However, Nutrasweet (aspertame) and Sweet'N Low (saccharin) are OK.

Raspberries (or Strawberries) and Cream

If you must have berries for dessert, use raspberries because they have the highest fiber content of all berries. If you simply don't like raspberries, strawberries are also relatively high in fiber content. Try to avoid even the berries for dessert if you have just consumed a large meal centered around red meats. For cream, use real cream or half and half instead of sugared whipped creams.

Goochi Apples

2 Golden Delicious apples, skin on, cut in
   chunks
1 small can unsweetened pineapple chunks (in
   own juice)
Handful of grapes
1 fresh satsuma orange, peeled and sectioned
   (optional)
$\frac{1}{2}$ cup orange juice
A few dashes of cinnamon
A few slivers of butter

In ovenproof dish, place apple chunks, pineapple with its own juice, grapes, satsuma sections, and orange juice. Sprinkle with cinnamon and a few slivers of butter, stir, cover, and bake in a pre-heated 350-degree oven for 20 minutes. This is not a particularly low-glycemic dessert, but it is a good one and may be eaten occasionally.

Serves 4.

XVI | Great New Orleans Restaurants Do SUGAR BUSTERS!

Now lets move to some of the SUGAR BUST-
ERS!–allowed recipes offered by outstanding
restaurants in New Orleans. You might remember, however, that Louisiana cooking has long
been scrutinized for its negative effects on health.
A national study has identified the area to be
densely populated with overweight citizens who
exhibit a high rate of heart disease, diabetes, and
other weight-related illnesses. Louisianians don't
eat to live, they live to eat.

What can be done about a tradition so ingrained? SUGAR BUSTERS! Many locals have
not only adopted the SUGAR BUSTERS! lifestyle,
but also converted and adhered to it with cultish
tenacity. People throughout the city are now getting slim! How can they give up their good old

New Orleans cuisine? Hey, they don't have to give it up. As you could see from the list in Figure 10 (pages 123–126), you can eat the likes of oysters, crawfish, steak, cheese, and on and on.

Many New Orleans restaurants now advertise SUGAR BUSTERS! dishes on their menus. It is not difficult to adapt most cuisine to the SUGAR BUSTERS! formula for healthy eating. Brown rice can be substituted for white rice. Stone-ground wheat bread can be substituted for white bread in dressings to impart a flavor that actually requires less seasoning. Sicilians traditionally add baking soda to tomato sauce instead of sugar to eliminate the acidic taste.

We wish to thank the talented chefs from famous New Orleans restaurants who have kindly agreed to share the following recipe collection with our readers. The recipes are the exclusive property of these restaurants or chefs.

From the kitchen of <u>Andrea's</u>

Whole-Wheat Pasta

Making Your Own Pasta

I highly recommend that you invest in a small pasta machine for your kitchen and make your own fresh pasta. It is no more difficult than making any other kind of dough, and it gives superior results. Although there are many complicated pasta machines on the market, the best gadget for making pasta is hand operated and very simple. A good pasta maker will be made of stainless steel and consists of a set of gear-driven rollers, about six inches long. By varying the space between the rollers, you control the thickness of the pasta. Regardless of the shape you will ultimately make your pasta into, here is the recipe for making the dough:

2 cups whole-wheat flour (preferably stone-
    ground)
1 whole egg

$^1/_2$ cup water

$^1/_2$ tsp. salt

1 tsp. extra virgin olive oil

Put the whole-wheat flour into the mixing bowl. Add the egg, water, salt, and oil and mix until firm. With your hands knead until you have a ball of dough (you may use a KitchenAid food processor to make it easier). *Note:* If the dough will not form a ball, add two tablespoons of water until it doesn't stick to your hands. Let the ball of dough sit covered with a towel for 10 minutes. Cut off a piece of dough about the size of your fist. Flatten it into a disk and dust lightly with flour. Set the dial on the pasta machine at 1, the thickest setting. Run the disk of pasta dough through. Dust it with flour, fold it over end to end, and run it through again. Change the setting to 3, and repeat the above procedure. Set the machine to 5, and go through the procedure yet again. By now, you should have a long strip of pasta. (Catch the end of the pasta with your free hand and pull it away as it exits the machine, so it does not pile up.) Change the setting to 6, the thinnest setting, and run through once more, but don't fold it over this time.

You now have a basic flat pasta sheet. You can use the attachments that come with the machine to cut it into angel hair, spaghetti, linguine, or fettuccine. Makes four 4-oz. portions (appetizer or side dish) or two 8-oz. portions (entrée size). Serve with two cups of Salsa Pomidoro Basilico (tomato basil sauce; see following recipe).

Salsa Pomidoro Basilico

1 tbsp. olive oil
$1/8$ cup chopped onion
1 tsp. chopped garlic
$1/4$ cup red wine
2 cups canned Italian plum tomatoes (check for no added sugar)
2 cups juice from tomatoes
$1/2$ tsp. salt
$1/4$ tsp. white pepper
2 sprigs chopped fresh oregano
8 chopped fresh basil leaves

4 chopped sprigs Italian parsley
1 bay leaf

In a saucepan over medium heat, heat the olive oil until very hot. In it sauté the onions and garlic until they are transparent. Add wine and bring to a boil. Immediately add the tomatoes, squeezing them between your fingers to break them up as you add them. Add tomato juice. Lower the heat and simmer the sauce. After about 30 minutes, add water (1 cup or less) if necessary to give the sauce the right consistency. You want the sauce thin enough to be able to easily coat the pasta, yet not so thin that it runs off the pasta. Add salt, pepper, oregano, basil, parsley, and bay leaf. Simmer sauce another 15 to 20 minutes. Adjust seasonings as needed. Makes about 1 quart, enough for about 8 pasta entrées.

Variation: You can add 5 shrimp per portion if you desire to use with the pasta. The sauce also can be used on chicken breast, beef, turkey, and veal.

Dentice in Acqua Pazza (Red Snapper in Crazy Water)

Red snapper is rightly one of the most celebrated denizens of the Gulf waters, but for some reason it is not frequently served outside New Orleans. I buy it whenever I can get it fresh. This dish is finished in a rather wet sauce. Its steaming effect makes the fillet extremely moist, but not mushy.

2 tbsp. extra virgin olive oil
2 cloves garlic, lightly crushed to break skin
1 tsp. red pepper flakes, crushed
4 red snapper fillets, 4 to 6 oz. each
1 cup canned Italian plum tomatoes, chopped
2 cups fish stock (can use clam juice)
1/2 tsp. salt
Pinch of white pepper
3 sprigs fresh oregano leaves

Preheat oven to 400 degrees. Heat olive oil in a skillet over high heat. Sauté garlic cloves until they begin to brown around the edges. Add crushed red pepper. Put two fish fillets at a time into the hot skillet, and sauté 30 seconds on each side. Remove from pan and keep warm. Add the tomatoes, fish stock, salt, pepper, and oregano to the skillet and bring to a boil over high heat. Lower the heat to medium and simmer the sauce for 5 minutes. Put the fish back in the skillet, and put the skillet into the oven for about 5 minutes until fish is cooked. (Don't use a skillet with a wooden or plastic handle!) Spoon sauce over fish and serve with a sprig of fresh oregano.

Serves 4.

From the kitchen of <u>Antoine's</u>

Filet de Boeuf Nature Marchand de Vin (Filet with Marchand de Vin Sauce)

Filet

Four 10-oz. beef tenderloins
1 tbsp. olive oil
Salt and pepper to taste
1 tbsp. chopped parsley for garnish

Brush the filets with the oil and season the meat with salt and pepper. Cook on a grill or heavy iron skillet, first on one side then the other, to desired doneness. Place filet in the middle of the plate, topped with Marchand de Vin sauce (see following recipe). Sprinkle top with chopped parsley.

Serves 4.

Roux

4 tbsp. melted butter
4 tbsp. whole-wheat flour

Sauce

1 cup chopped white onion
1 cup chopped mushrooms
6 cloves minced garlic
3 tbsp. butter
2 cups beef stock (salt and pepper to taste)
1 cup red wine
3 tbsp. Lea & Perrins Worcestershire sauce
Salt and pepper to taste

For the roux, in a small heavy skillet melt butter and add the flour. Brown flour until it becomes a dark caramel color and set aside. For the sauce, sauté the onions, mushrooms, and garlic with butter until lightly browned. Add the beef stock, wine, Lea & Perrins Worcestershire sauce, and salt and pepper. Cook for 15 minutes, reducing the liquid, and then add the roux. Mix well.

Makes about 3 cups.

Shrimp Ravigote

6 leaves lettuce
2 cups shredded lettuce
6 tomatoes, each cut into 6 wedges
2 lbs. boiled shrimp, peeled
1 cup Ravigote sauce (see following recipe)
6 anchovy filets
Vinaigrette (see following recipe)

Place a green leaf in the center of the plate. Put 1/3 cup of shredded lettuce in the center of the leaf. Place a tomato wedge on each side of the leaf. Mix peeled shrimp into Ravigote sauce. Put 6 oz. of shrimp Ravigote on each plate and top with anchovy filet. Pour 1 oz. of vinaigrette over the top.

Serves 6.

Ravigote Sauce

1½ cups mayonnaise
1½ tbsp. minced bell pepper
1½ tbsp. minced green onions
1½ tbsp. minced anchovies
1½ tbsp. minced pimento

Mix all ingredients together and chill.

Vinaigrette Sauce

1 cup olive oil
⅓ cup vinegar

$^1/_2$ tsp. dry powdered mustard
$^1/_2$ tsp. salt
$^1/_2$ tsp. finely ground white pepper

Put all ingredients into a bottle and shake to mix.

From the kitchen of <u>Bacco</u>

Chicken Cacciatore

$3^1/_2$ lb. roasting chicken, skinned and cut into
   8 pieces
1 large clove garlic, minced
3-inch piece of fresh rosemary
$^1/_4$ tsp. salt
4 tbsp. extra virgin olive oil
$^1/_4$ tsp. fresh ground black pepper
3 red bell peppers cut into 1-inch triangles
$^1/_4$ cup chopped onions
$^1/_2$ cup canned plum tomatoes
$^1/_2$ cup red wine
1 qt. chicken stock
salt and pepper

Rinse and dry the chicken pieces. Combine the garlic, rosemary, and salt in a food processor and crush into a paste. Rub the paste into the chicken pieces, cover with plastic wrap and refrigerate for 24 hours. Heat the oil in a sauté pan over medium-high heat. Brown the chicken pieces until golden on all sides. Sprinkle with black pepper while browning. Remove chicken from pan and set aside. Add the peppers and onions. Cook until onions become translucent and add the chicken back to the pan, add the tomatoes and the red wine. Cook about 20 minutes, until wine evaporates. Add chicken stock and simmer for another 20 minutes over medium-low heat or until chicken is tender. Add salt and pepper to taste before serving. Serve in a large warmed bowl with a thick slice of grilled whole-wheat bread rubbed with a fresh clove of garlic.

Serves 2.

Gulf Shrimp and Whole-Wheat Linguine

1 oz. olive oil
1 oz. slivered garlic

8 shrimp, peeled, deveined, tail on

1/4 tsp. crushed red pepper

1/4 cup white wine

1/4 oz. fresh basil

4 oz. bitter greens (rapini) raw, torn into smaller
pieces

4 oz. whole-wheat linguine (cooked al dente)

1 tbsp. extra virgin olive oil

salt and black pepper to taste

In a medium sauté pan heat olive oil and garlic together over medium-high heat until garlic is browned. This must constantly be stirred while garlic is browning. Once garlic is browned add shrimp, salt, pepper and crushed red pepper. Sauté for about 1–2 minutes. Add white wine, fresh basil, bitter greens and 2–3 oz. of water. Cook over high heat until shrimp are cooked. Add cooked and heated linguine to sauté pan, and toss well with shrimp mixture and extra virgin olive oil. Salt and pepper to taste. Place in pasta bowl and drizzle small amount of olive oil over the top. Garnish with a fresh basil flower.

Chef's Note: Correctly browning the slivered garlic is a very important step in this dish because all of the flavor comes from the garlic. Be careful to brown the garlic, not burn it. If any of the garlic is burned it will make the dish bitter.

Serves 2.

From the kitchen of <u>Bella Luna</u>

Confit of Duck

12 duck legs or 3 duck breasts cut into thick
  strips
3 cloves minced garlic
1 cup chopped celery
1 cup chopped onion
1/4 cup fresh, chopped herbs (thyme, rosemary,
  oregano)
1 cup dark stock (see following recipe)
1 cup Merlot wine
Salt and pepper to taste

Place duck in skillet over medium heat and sear until brown. Remove from the skillet and hold on the side. Add garlic, celery, onion, and herbs to the skillet and sauté 4 to 5 minutes. Place the duck on top of the herbs and onions. Add stock and wine and simmer in oven at 375 degrees for 2½ to 3 hours; test with a knife to make sure the meat is done. The meat should fall off the bone. You may need to add water and/or wine during the cooking time. Remove duck from sauce, strain the herbs, celery, and onions from the sauce, and skim off the fat from the top. Next, cut off the extra fat and skin from the duck. Pour the sauce over the meat and serve with brown rice.

Serves 4.

Dark Stock

2 lbs. bones (beef or pork)
2 onions, sliced
2 cloves garlic, minced
3 sticks celery, diced
Red wine
½ cup fresh rosemary, thyme, and oregano

For dark stock, roast bones in deep roasting pan with onions, garlic, and celery until browned. Deglaze with red wine several times during roasting. When the color is right (dark), add cold water to cover. Add herbs for seasoning. Simmer on stove for 4 to 5 hours until dark and concentrated. Strain before using. Stock can be frozen for later use.

Venison Tenderloin in Beer Glaze

One 16-oz. venison tenderloin (backstrap)
Salt and pepper to taste
Ground cloves to taste
2 tbsp. butter
Rosemary and thyme, fresh
3 cloves garlic
1 cup dark stock (recipe on page 214)
1/2 cup beer

Season tenderloin with salt, pepper, and ground cloves. Sear tenderloin in butter on all sides over medium heat, then add herbs and garlic and finish in oven for 10 minutes at 375 degrees. After 10 minutes, take the pan out of oven, remove the venison, and deglaze skillet with dark stock and beer. Reduce for 5 minutes on the burner over medium heat. Strain the herbs from the sauce. Slice venison tenderloin, put on plate, and lightly cover with sauce.

Serves 4.

From the kitchen of <u>Commander's Palace Restaurant</u>

Grilled Filet of Beef

8 oz. filet of beef
Kosher salt and cracked black pepper
3 oz. asparagus
1 tbsp. butter
2 oz. water
4 oz. roasted sweet potatoes
2 oz. Hollandaise sauce (see following recipe)

Season filet with kosher salt and pepper on both sides. Grill over hickory to your temperature (preferred doneness). Steam asparagus in medium sauté pan with butter and water. Salt and pepper to taste.

Roast sweet potatoes with skin on in oven at 350 degrees until a fork or knife goes through. Peel the skin from the potatoes.

Place filet on plate. Place steamed asparagus to one side of the filet and arrange peeled sliced sweet potatoes on the other. Top filet with Hollandaise.

Serves 1.

Hollandaise Sauce

1 egg yolk
1/2 lemon, juice only
Salt and white pepper to taste
1 1/2 oz. clarified butter (melted and skimmed)
1 tbsp. water

This can easily be burned if not heated properly. Fill a saucepan or Dutch oven large enough to accommodate the mixing bowl with about 1 inch of water. Heat the water to just below the boiling point. Place the egg yolk, lemon juice, salt, and white pepper in the mixing bowl. Set the bowl in the pan over the water; do not let the water touch the bottom of the bowl. Whisk the egg yolk mixture until slightly thickened, then drizzle the clarified butter into the yolk, whisking constantly. If the bottom of the bowl becomes hotter than warm to the touch, remove the bowl from the pan of water for a few seconds and let cool. When all of the butter is incorporated and the sauce is thick, beat in the tablespoon of water. Serve the Hollandaise immediately or keep in a warm place at room temperature until time to use.

Yields 2 cups.

Hickory-Grilled Shrimp with Summer Green Salad

Six 15- to 20-count fresh shrimp
½ oz. olive oil
1 tsp. fresh garlic
1 tbsp. fresh herbs, finely chopped (rosemary, oregano, and basil)
Kosher salt and black pepper to taste
3 tomato slices, creole or vine-ripe

4 oz. baby greens

1/2 cucumber, peeled, seeded, then sliced

1 oz. cane vinaigrette (see following recipe)

3 thin slices red onion

1/2 oz. hard goat cheese, grated

Marinate shrimp with olive oil, garlic, fresh herbs, salt, and pepper for 1/2 hour. Then grill over hickory. Place 3 tomato slices on a plate at the top. Season with kosher salt and black pepper. Toss baby greens and cucumber with cane vinaigrette. Place in the center of the plate beside the tomatoes. Place shrimp on top of greens and garnish with sliced onions and grated goat cheese.

Serves 1.

Cane Vinaigrette

1 oz. cane vinegar

1 oz. extra virgin olive oil

1 tsp. dry mustard

1 tsp. fresh basil

Salt and pepper to taste

Mix all ingredients.

From the kitchen of <u>Croziers</u>

Lamb Loin Provençale

8 lamb tenderloins cut in half (or 8 lamb chops)
2 tsp. Dijon mustard
1 tsp. finely chopped fresh rosemary
6 tbsp. olive oil
4 tomatoes
Salt and pepper
6 tbsp. bread crumbs (preferably whole-grain)
2 tbsp. chopped parsley
1 tsp. chopped garlic
1 tsp. fresh thyme or 1/2 tsp. dried thyme
1/2 to 3/4 cup inexpensive dry white wine

Salt and pepper the tenderloins. Mix the mustard with chopped rosemary and 2 tbsp. of olive oil, and place the tenderloins in this marinade for 1/2 hour to 1 hour. Meanwhile, halve the tomatoes and sprinkle with salt and pepper. Mix the bread crumbs with the parsley, garlic, and thyme, and divide this mixture equally on top of tomato halves. Sprinkle a little olive oil on top. Place in ovenproof dish coated with a bit of oil, and cook in 425-degree oven for 30 minutes. When tomatoes are ready, remove the lamb from marinade, scraping most of the marinade off, and sauté in hot oil until brown on all sides and of desired doneness. It will take 4 to 5 minutes altogether depending on the thickness of the meat. Remove meat from pan and pour off any grease. Then add 1/2 cup wine to pan, scraping any brown bits accumulated in bottom of pan, into the wine. Remove from heat, and if any natural juices have seeped from the meat, add to the sauce, mix, and pour over the meat. Surround with baked tomato halves. Sprinkle with extra chopped parsley if desired.

Serves 4.

Sweet Potatoes Lyonnaise

2 large sweet potatoes, baked until still slightly
   firm, cooled, and peeled
Olive oil
1 medium onion
Salt and pepper to taste

Slice the sweet potatoes in thick slices, and sauté in 2 tbsp. olive oil, peanut oil, or butter until slightly browned. Slice the onion in thin slices, and sauté in 1 tbsp. olive oil, peanut oil, or butter until lightly browned. Combine onions and sweet potatoes and sprinkle with salt and pepper to taste (don't overdo the portions of this dish).

Serves 4.

From the kitchen of <u>Emeril's Restaurant</u>

Emeril's Pan-roasted Filet Mignon Stuffed with Maytag Blue Cheese Served with a Warm Haricot Vert and Bacon Salad

1/2 lb. bacon, chopped
1 cup julienned yellow onions
1 tsp. chopped garlic
1/2 cup walnut pieces
1 lb. green beans, blanched and shocked in ice
    water
Salt and black pepper

Four 8-oz. filet mignons
1 cup crumbled Maytag blue cheese
Salt and cracked pepper
2 tbsp. olive oil
1 tbsp. chopped parsley

Preheat the oven to 400 degrees. In a hot sauté pan, render the bacon until crispy, stirring occasionally, about 8 minutes. Stir in the onions, garlic, and walnuts. Sauté for 3 minutes. Add the green beans. Season with salt and pepper. Sauté for 2 minutes. Reduce heat to low to keep the salad warm. On the side of each filet make a 2-inch slit forming a pocket. Stuff each pocket with 2 tbsp. of the cheese. Season the filets with salt and cracked pepper. In ovenproof sauté pan, add the olive oil. When the oil is hot, sear the filets for 2 minutes on each side. Place the pan in the oven and roast the filets for 6 to 7 minutes for medium-rare. Remove filets from the pan. To serve, spoon the salad into the center of each plate. Place the filets on top of the salad. Garnish with parsley.

Serves 4 (main course).

Emeril's Bouillabaisse

2 tbsp. olive oil
1 cup chopped onion
1/2 cup chopped celery
3 cloves garlic
1 bay leaf
8 black peppercorns
2 sprigs thyme
1 lb. fish bones
Water to cover
1 cup white wine
Pinch of saffron
1 cup julienned leeks
3 cups peeled, seeded, and chopped tomatoes
Juice and zest of one orange
1 cup julienned fennel
2 tbsp. chopped garlic
2 tbsp. finely chopped parsley
2 lbs. assorted small, whole, fresh trout, perch, or
    farm-raised catfish, cleaned and scaled
1 large lobster
1 lb. shrimp, peeled and deveined
1/2 lb. littleneck clams
1/2 lb. mussels

Salt and pepper to taste
Rouille (see following recipe)

For the stock, in a large saucepan, heat the olive oil. Add the onions and celery. Season with salt and pepper. Sauté for 3 minutes. Add 3 cloves garlic and cook for 1 minute. Add the bay leaf, peppercorns, and thyme. Add the fish bones, water to cover, and wine. Bring the liquid to a boil and reduce to a simmer. Cook for 30 minutes. Remove from the heat and strain.

For the bouillabaisse, place the stock on the heat and bring to a simmer. Add the saffron, leeks, tomatoes, orange juice, orange zest, fennel, 2 tbsp. chopped garlic, and parsley. Season with salt and pepper. Add the fish and lobster. Cook for 8 minutes. Add the shrimp, clams, and mussels. Cook for 6 minutes, or until the shells have opened. Discard any shellfish that do not open. Season with salt and pepper. To assemble, arrange the seafood in a shallow dish. Ladle the stock over the seafood. Drizzle the rouille over the seafood.

Serves 6.

Rouille

1 red pepper, roasted and peeled
2 cloves garlic
1 egg yolk
1 tbsp. Dijon mustard
Juice of one lemon
3/4 cup olive oil
Salt and pepper

In a food processor, purée the first five ingredients until smooth. With the machine running, add the olive oil in a steady stream. Season the mixture with salt and pepper.

Yields about 1 cup.

From the kitchen of Galatoire's Restaurant

Crabmeat Yvonne

1 lb. fresh white mushrooms or Portabella
    mushrooms, sliced

1/2 cup clarified butter (melt in saucepan and
   skim off any milk solids)
6 fresh artichoke bottoms, boiled and sliced
2 lbs. fresh backfin lump crabmeat (Gulf of
   Mexico blue crabs)
Salt and white pepper to taste
Parsley, chopped fine

In a large skillet sauté the mushrooms in the butter, then add the artichoke bottoms and crabmeat.
Sauté gently until heated thoroughly. Season
with salt and white pepper. Garnish with finely
chopped parsley. Serve over toast points and with
a lemon wedge.

Serves 6.

Shrimp Remoulade

1 bunch green onions
2 stalks celery
3 cloves garlic
1 bunch parsley, stems removed
1 cup creole mustard

4 tbsp. paprika

2 tbsp. prepared horseradish

1 tsp. Tabasco

1 tsp. Worcestershire sauce

Salt and black pepper to taste, and pinch cayenne
    pepper

2/3 cup red wine vinegar

1 1/2 cups olive oil

2 1/2 lbs. shrimp, boiled, peeled, and deveined

1 head shredded lettuce

Chop onions, celery, garlic, and parsley very fine.
Remove to a ceramic or glass bowl and add creole
mustard, paprika, horseradish, Tabasco, Worcestershire sauce, salt and black pepper, and cayenne
pepper. Add red wine vinegar and gradually add
olive oil while whisking.

Fold in shrimp and let marinate several hours
or overnight in refrigerator. Serve cold over shredded lettuce.

6 appetizer size servings.

From the kitchen of <u>Mosca's</u>

Mosca's Chicken à la Grande

3/4 cup Bertolli olive oil
Two 3-lb. chickens (cut into eighths)
1/2 tsp. salt
1 tsp. freshly ground black pepper
10 cloves unpeeled garlic, mashed
1 tsp. rosemary
1 tsp. oregano
1 cup dry white wine

In a large skillet, heat the olive oil until it is hot and add the chicken pieces. Turn the chicken often, cooking until all pieces are browned. Sprinkle the chicken with salt and pepper. Add the garlic, rosemary, and oregano, stirring to distribute the seasonings. Pour the wine over the chicken, and simmer until the wine is reduced by half. Serve the chicken hot with the pan juices.

Serves 6.

Mosca's Italian Shrimp

2 lbs. large, whole fresh shrimp (with heads, in
   shells)
1 cup olive oil
1 tbsp. plus 1 tsp. salt
2 tsp. freshly ground black pepper
2 tsp. oregano leaves
2 tsp. rosemary leaves
3 bay leaves
25 cloves garlic, moderately mashed
1 cup dry white wine

Many chefs cook some variation of what New Or-
leanians refer to as barbeque shrimp. Nobody
makes an olive oil, garlic, oregano, and rosemary
version that's as good as Mosca's.

Place all the ingredients except the wine in a large
skillet, and cook over medium-high heat for 15 to
20 minutes or until the shrimp are pink and the
liquid produced by the shrimp has almost completely disappeared. Stir occasionally. Reduce the
heat and add the wine. Cook at a low simmer until the liquid is reduced by half, about 5 to 7 min-

utes. Serve the shrimp hot with the pan juices. A good whole-grain bread for dipping is a nice accompaniment.

Serves 6.

From the kitchen of the <u>Palace Cafe</u>

Pasta St. Charles

4 tbsp. butter
12 oz. andouille or another heavily smoked
  sausage, sliced, then cut in half
2 tbsp. garlic, minced
2 bunches green onions, sliced (put aside 2 tbsp.
  green onions, minced for garnish)
2 oz. white wine
1 lb. shrimp (36–42 count), peeled and deveined
2 tbsp. creole mustard
12 oz. heavy cream
1/2 lb. whole-grain wheat penne pasta, cooked
Salt and pepper
2 oz. Parmesan cheese

In a medium to large sauté pan, melt 2 tbsp. butter. Over medium-high heat, add andouille sausage and sauté for 1 minute. Add garlic and green onions, and sauté for 1 minute. Add white wine, reduce by half, and add shrimp and creole mustard. Add cream and reduce by one third. Add pasta. Toss and season with salt and pepper. Add remaining butter, and separate into 4 bowls. Garnish with green onions and Parmesan cheese.

Serves 4.

SUGAR BUSTERS! *Salad*

2/3 cup very coarse bulgur wheat (dry)

1 1/2 cups chick peas (cooked, strained, and chilled)

1/3 cup orange lentils (dry) or similar (French lentils)

1/3 cup chopped green onions

1 1/2 cups chopped Roma tomato

1 1/2 cup finely chopped parsley

1 cup crumbled feta cheese

3/4 cup extra virgin olive oil

1 cup fresh lemon juice (or to taste)
Salt and pepper to taste

Rinse and drain bulgur wheat three times. Then soak in warm water and set aside. Next, rinse lentils thoroughly. Simmer in water or chicken broth until tender. Do not overcook. Immediately drain lentils and rinse with cold water. In large mixing bowl, add remaining ingredients. Mix, then add bulgur wheat and lentils. Taste and season. Water or more oil may be needed as lentils and wheat soak up juices. Serve at room temperature. Store in refrigerator. When serving, liquids may need to be added again.

Serves 8.

From the kitchen of <u>Upperline Restaurant</u>

Chilled Creole Tomato Soup with Crab Guacamole

1 oz. olive oil
1 small leek, rinsed and sliced

1 small white onion, sliced
1 red bell pepper, sliced and deseeded
1/2 tsp. crushed garlic
1 rib celery, sliced
4 large ripe creole tomatoes (diced)
2 cups chicken stock
1/8 tsp. pepper flakes
Salt and pepper to taste
Crab guacamole (see following recipe)

In medium saucepan, heat olive oil and simmer the leek, onion, red bell pepper, garlic, and celery 10 minutes over medium heat. Do not brown. Add tomatoes, chicken stock, and pepper flakes, and simmer 30 minutes. Season with salt and pepper. Purée in food processor (do not strain). Cool and serve. Garnish soup with crab guacamole.

Serves 4.

Crab Guacamole

1 ripe avocado
1 lime

Salt to taste

4 oz. bluepoint crabmeat (Gulf of Mexico)

Mash avocado meat, and season with lime juice and salt. Fold in crabmeat; garnish soup.

Serves 4.

Grilled Portobello Mushrooms with Brown Rice and Goat Cheese

1 cup brown rice

3 cups chicken stock

Dressing (see following recipe)

1/2 tsp. salt

4 medium-size Portobello mushroom caps

1 oz. extra virgin olive oil

Salt and pepper to taste

2 oz. goat cheese (at room temperature)

First prepare the brown rice by combining the rice and chicken stock in a medium saucepan. Simmer for 1 hour or until the rice is tender. You may need to add more stock if necessary. Season, strain out extra stock, and let cool. Mix cooked rice with dressing. Reserve. To cook the mushrooms, remove the large stem. Brush oil on gill side of mushrooms, and season with salt and pepper. Have grill on medium heat. Place mushrooms gill side down, and cook 2 minutes. Flip over, and cook 2 more minutes. (Be sure not to burn; flip and move constantly so that the mushrooms cook through evenly.) When the mushrooms are tender and flexible, they are ready. Remove and either slice them or leave whole. Keep warm. Place brown rice salad on the plate. Put the mushrooms over that and top with dabs of goat cheese. Enjoy!

Serves 2.

Dressing

1 tsp. Dijon mustard (or no-sugar mustard)
3 tbsp. sherry vinegar
6 tbsp. olive oil
Chopped fresh tarragon

Put mustard in a salad bowl, then whisk in vinegar, then oil, then herbs.

From the kitchen of the <u>Windsor Court Hotel</u>

Marinated Portobello Mushroom Salad with Stilton Cheese and Bacon

2 Portobello mushrooms
6 oz. olive oil
3 oz. red wine vinegar
1/2 oz. soy sauce
1 clove garlic
2 oz. mixed greens
2 slices bacon, fried crisp
1 oz. Stilton or another blue cheese

Clean two stemless Portobellos with damp rag. Blend 4 oz. oil, 2 oz. vinegar, soy sauce, and garlic, and pour over mushroom caps. Let sit overnight.

Mix greens with 2 oz. olive oil and 1 oz. red wine vinegar, then toss. Top with diced crisp bacon and crumbled cheese. Grill Portobellos 4 to 5 minutes. Top salad with warm mushrooms.

Serves 2.

SUGAR BUSTERS! *Chocolate Mousse*

1$\frac{1}{2}$ lbs. chocolate (must be at least 60 percent cocoa)
1$\frac{1}{2}$ qts. heavy cream
5 egg yolks
6 oz. decaffeinated coffee
5 egg whites

Melt chocolate in microwave or over boiling water. Boil 2 cups cream. Add egg yolks and decaffeinated coffee, then pour boiled cream over chocolate. Whisk until no lumps remain. Whip egg whites and fold into mousse. Whip 1 qt. cream to soft peaks, then fold into mousse. Chill until ready to serve.

Serves 8–10.

XVII|Frequently Asked Questions

After two years of responses to the Voluntary Mailback Questionnaire in the back of the original SUGAR BUSTERS! and also following a year of screening questions from our Web Site, we have included answers for the most commonly asked questions. The most frequent information requests have been addressed in the new Fourteen-Day Meal Plan, the Recipe chapter, and the expanded Glycemic index in Figure 4 (pages 61–65).

The response to the original SUGAR BUSTERS! was overwhelming regarding weight loss and improved blood chemistries. For those of you whose questions we simply could not address in a timely manner, we apologize and hope that you will find your questions answered in this chapter.

Q. What kind of breads can I eat?

A. Whole-grain breads without a significant amount of added sugar, molasses, etc. Next best are stone-ground whole-wheat breads without the sugars.

Q. How much of an allowed bread can I eat?

A. Two slices daily if you wish to lose weight. Three slices maximum on a maintenance program.

Q. Can I truly eat large amounts of proteins?

A. No, portion size is important; excess protein is converted to fat and can cause weight gain in some people.

Q. When you eat a high-fat meal, should you eliminate nearly all carbohydrates?

A. One should *not* eat a high-fat meal. Fat primarily should be consumed in combination with lean, trimmed meats, or mono- or poly-unsaturated oils. If you must eat a high-fat meal, combine it only with low-glycemic carbohydrates.

Q. What fruit juices are best to drink?

A. Those that are unsweetened. Better are those that are freshly squeezed from the whole fruit. Best yet would be to eat the whole fruit itself.

Fruit drinks and "sport drinks" are not accept-able as they have excessive amounts of added refined sugar.

Q. Most "no-sugar-added" foods contain ingredi-ents such as maltodextrin, malted barley, poly-dextrose, maltitol, sorbitol, or sugar alcohol. Which ones, if any, are OK?

A. They are all carbohydrates and, as such, ele-vate the blood sugar. However, their glycemic index is much lower than that of glucose. They should be consumed in as small amounts as possible.

Q. Is food starch or cornstarch OK?

A. No, starch is simply a large sugar molecule. Once in our digestive tracts, starch quickly be-comes glucose.

Q. Do any vitamin pills cause significant insulin secretion since some contain sugar or food starch?

A. No, the sugar coating or fills are only a mini-mal amount of sugar.

Q. How or when do high levels of circulating fat get reduced or eliminated when there is little insulin present in your system?

A. Fat is converted by hormone-sensitive lipase

to free fatty acids that are burned as energy sources by many of our vital organs, such as the heart, kidneys, and muscle.

Q. Why does the SUGAR BUSTERS! lifestyle cause triglyceride levels to drop?

A. By reducing sugar and insulin. Remember that insulin facilitates the conversion of excess sugar to fat and triglycerides are fat.

Q. What is happening that allows slim, middle-aged people to consume huge quantities of sugar or high-glycemic carbohydrates and not have it deposited as fat?

A. Some individuals have a higher metabolic rate and/or more muscle mass, which utilizes most consumed sugar as an energy source. Therefore, very little sugar remains for conversion to fat.

Q. What are people's most common problems in not achieving weight loss on the SUGAR BUSTERS! lifestyle?

A. First, eating too much of a "legal" carbohydrate like whole-wheat breads and pastas, sweet potatoes, etc. Second, too much snacking and/or cheating, although modestly, too frequently. Third, not exercising. Fourth, genetic predisposition to store fat. Fifth, supplemental hormones.

Q. Where can I find high-cocoa-content chocolate?

A. Le Noir American Chocolate, which is available in many stores and contains 71% cocoa. Also, Valvrona makes a high-cocoa chocolate that is distributed in the United States.

Q. How many grams of refined sugar can or should be consumed per day?

A. None would be preferred but certainly as few as possible. Any single food source, such as cereal, should contain 3 grams or less.

Q. What is the difference between whole-wheat, whole-grain, and stone-ground wheat? Are all acceptable breads?

A. Basically they are all the same, except whole grain may contain grains other than wheat, such as oats or rye. The problem exists with the amount of sugars the manufacturer may have added and the degree of refining (particle size) of the flour. The coarser, the better.

Q. Why do you list shredded wheat and rice cakes as allowed to eat on your sample meal plan (in your original book)?

A. Nabisco/Post Original Shredded Wheat 'N Bran and brown (inadvertently omitted) rice cakes are allowed because their glycemic indexes are lower than for "white" versions.

Q. If a high-cocoa-content chocolate (which still contains refined sugar) is acceptable as a mid-afternoon snack, why may I not eat a banana just as well?

A. One may. However, both are higher glycemic snacks than a Triscuit with a slim layer of cheese or a lower glycemic fruit, such as an apple, pear, or orange.

Q. What ice creams or yogurts are acceptable?

A. Low-fat, no-added-sugar types are the best. However, none are good choices if too frequently consumed when you wish to lose weight.

Q. Is high-fructose corn syrup OK?

A. No, it is a high-glycemic sweetener.

Q. Is semolina flour OK?

A. Yes, it is the remaining flour particles after the fine, white component has been removed. But it should not have been additionally processed.

Q. Is whole milk OK to drink?

A. Skimmed or 2% contains less butter (fat); 2%

is a good compromise between skimmed and whole milk.

Q. Are all nuts OK, and are seeds (pumpkin or sunflower) OK?

A. Yes, but again in moderation, only a few at a time. No more than a dozen.

Q. Is blue corn OK?

A. No.

Q. Is salt OK?

A. Preferably no added salt at the table. Only use lightly as seasoning when cooking as too much salt can cause you to retain water; therefore, salt is a leading contributor to high blood pressure.

Q. Are grits and couscous OK?

A. Grits are not OK because they are made from ground corn. Couscous is OK only if it is whole-wheat couscous.

Q. Are yams and sweet potatoes the same?

A. Not technically, but for all practical purposes, in the United States they are the same.

Q. Why are sugar-free pudding and Jell-O not OK?

A. They are OK, especially those that are also fat free.

Q. Is Coffeemate allowed?

A. No, it contains coconut oil, which is high in cholesterol.

Q. May I have fruit with a meal if it does not cause me to have indigestion?

A. Yes. However, fruit ideally should be consumed by itself as a snack to receive the best benefit of lower insulin secretion after a meal. Also, many people have improved digestion by consuming fruit thirty minutes before or two hours after a meal.

Q. Is the SUGAR BUSTERS! lifestyle good for children?

A. Yes; over 50% of children are overweight, and this is primarily from too much sugar. In addition, elevated insulin levels during childhood and young adulthood predispose one to an increased risk of obesity, diabetes, hypertension, and vascular diseases in later life.

Q. Is the SUGAR BUSTERS! lifestyle good for pregnant women?

A. Yes; by following the SUGAR BUSTERS! lifestyle women are less likely to be prediabetic or diabetic during pregnancy, which in turn reduces the incidence of diabetes in their children in later life.

Layman's Glossary

Amino acids   the building blocks of all protein. There are nine essential, or necessary, amino acids that the body cannot make itself and that must be provided from the foods we eat (an egg contains all nine).

Amylase   enzymes secreted by the salivary glands and the pancreas that break down carbohydrates.

Antioxidants   chemical compounds that readily accept an oxygen-free radical, thus inhibiting the oxidation of polyunsaturated fatty acids that are important to maintaining cellular health. Vitamins A, C, and E are antioxidants.

Atheroma   (also referred to as a *plaque*) a deposit of cholesterol, calcium, and blood clot in the lining of major vessels, eventually leading to blockage.

Arteriosclerosis   the process of hardening of arteries through the formation of plaques on the inner lining of major blood vessels.

Beta cells   specialized cells in the pancreas responsible for the production and secretion of insulin.

Bioflavonoids   compounds found in nature mostly as

yellow pigments that contain no nutritional value, but may help preserve the health of arterial walls by reducing their cholesterol content.

Blood clot   coagulated or congealed blood.

Calorie   The unit of heat energy required to raise 1 kilogram of water 1 degree Celsius.

Carbohydrates   chemical compounds containing carbon, hydrogen, and oxygen. Carbohydrates are a storage form of sugar.

Cholesterol   a compound belonging to a family of substances called sterols. It usually combines with fat when circulating in the bloodstream for distribution to all cells.

Complex carbohydrate   a carbohydrate with a more complex structure, such as starch or glycogen. The degree of complexity does not indicate the rate at which the carbohydrate is digested.

Diabetes mellitus, Type I   a disease characterized by the lack of insulin and the resulting elevated blood glucose (sugar) levels.

Diabetes mellitus, Type II   a disease characterized by resistance of the cells in the body to the actions of insulin and that also leads to elevated blood glucose (sugar) levels.

Energy   capacity to produce motion or heat.

Free fatty acid   the structural component of fat.

Fructose   a simple sugar found in fruits. Its insulin-stimulating effect is lower than that of galactose and glucose.

Galactose   a simple sugar found in dairy products. Its insulin-stimulating effect is less than glucose.

Gastric emptying the process of emptying food from the stomach or the time required to empty a meal from the stomach.

Glucagon hormone secreted by the pancreas that helps regulate blood sugar and metabolize stored fat.

Glucose the form in which sugar circulates in the bloodstream; the body's main energy source.

Glycemic index how rapidly a carbohydrate food is digested into glucose and how much it causes the blood sugar (glucose) to rise.

Glyceride a group name for fats. Mono-, di-, and triglycerides, which contain one, two, or three fatty acids, are the main constituents of fats.

Glycerol a constituent of fats. Chemically, it is an alcohol that combines with fatty acids to produce fats.

Glycerol-3-phosphate a metabolic product that occurs when glucose transforms into triglycerides.

Glycogen a complex form of glucose that is stored in the liver and muscle to be used to meet energy needs.

High-density lipoprotein (HDL) lipoproteins carrying cholesterol from the cells to the liver for breakdown and elimination from the body, probably the single best determinant of risk for coronary artery disease and heart attacks.

High-density lipoprotein (HDL) cholesterol high-density lipoprotein cholesterol thought to be protective against heart disease.

Hyperglycemia abnormally elevated blood glucose (sugar) level.

Hyperlipidemia abnormally elevated blood lipids, usually either cholesterol or triglycerides or both.

Hypertension   persistently elevated blood pressure.

Hypoglycemia   an abnormally low blood glucose (sugar) sugar level.

Insulin   hormone secreted by the pancreas. It lowers blood glucose by directing cells to utilize the glucose.

Insulin resistance   failure of insulin to exert its normal effect of allowing glucose into cells. This causes a rise in blood glucose (sugar) levels and therefore triggers the need for still more insulin.

Lipase   enzymes secreted by the pancreas that digest fats.

Lipid   a fat of either plant or animal origin.

Lipogenesis   the formation of fat from glucose.

Lipolysis   the breakdown of triglycerides to free fatty acids and glycerol, both of which are used as energy sources for the body.

Lipoproteins   combination of fat and proteins that circulate in the bloodstream. They function as the major carriers of lipids.

Lipoprotein lipase   a very important enzyme in the storage of fat.

Liver   a large organ that directs the metabolism of carbohydrates, proteins, and fats and the manufacture of enzymes, cholesterol, and other important substances. Our "metabolic computer."

Low-density lipoproteins (LDL)   lipoproteins that are important in the transport of cholesterol.

Low-density lipoprotein (LDL) cholesterol   low-density lipoprotein cholesterol, thought to be a major risk factor for heart disease.

Lymphatic system   vessels and lymph tissue that drain tissue fluid back into the cardiovascular system. It is the main route of absorption of fats from the small intestine.

Metabolism the sum of all the chemical and physiological processes by which the body grows and maintains itself and by which it breaks matter down into a new state.

Modulate regulate or control the flow of.

Monounsaturated fats fat molecules containing only one double bond. Examples are olives, peanuts, and pecans.

Obesity the presence of excess body fat.

Pancreas an important organ that produces both insulin and glucagon, as well as digestive enzymes such as lipase.

Plasma fibrinogen protein used in making blood clots.

Plaque deposits of cholesterol, calcium, and blood clot on the lining of major vessels. Also called *atheroma*.

Platelets elements in blood that are important in the clotting process by sticking to each other and starting the process of clot formation.

Polyunsaturated fats fat molecules containing two or more double bonds. Most vegetable oils are polyunsaturated.

Saturated fats fat molecules containing carbon atoms that are fully bound with hydrogen atoms such as most animal fats.

Simple sugars also known as *monosaccharides*. The most important are glucose, fructose (fruit sugar), and galactose (milk sugar).

Sterols complex steroids, one of which is cholesterol.

Syndrome X the combination of two or more of the following: insulin resistance, elevated insulin levels, elevated triglycerides, obesity, and hypertension.

Synthesis the manufacture or creation of a new substance.

Triglycerides the main type of stored fat in most animal systems.

Type I diabetes mellitus a disease characterized by the lack of insulin and the resulting elevated blood glucose (sugar) levels.

Type II diabetes mellitus a disease characterized by resistance of the cells in the body to the actions of insulin and that also leads to elevated blood glucose (sugar) levels.

Very low density lipoproteins (VLDL) lipoproteins that are important in transport of fatty components from the liver to fat cells.

References

Anderson, K. M., W. P. Castelli, and D. Levy. "Cholesterol and Mortality: 30 Years of Follow-Up from the Framingham Study." *Journal of the American Medical Association* 257 (1987): 2176–2180.

Artaud-Wild, S. M., S. L. Connor, G. Sexton, and W. E. Connor. "Differences in Coronary Mortality Can Be Explained by Differences in Cholesterol and Saturated Fat Intakes in 40 Countries but Not in France and Finland: A Paradox." *Circulation* 88 (1993): 2771–2779.

Brand, J. C., B. J. Snow, G. P. Nabhan, and A. S. Truswell. "Plasma Glucose and Insulin Responses to Traditional Pima Indian Meals." *American Journal of Clinical Nutrition* 51 (1990): 416–420.

Cowie, Catherine C., and Mark S. Eberhardt, eds. *Diabetes 1996: Vital Statistics.* 1996: 15, 16.

deLorgeril, M., N. Mamelle, and P. A. Salen. "A Mediterranean Type Diet in the Secondary Prevention of Coronary Heart Disease." *Circulation* 88 (Suppl.) (1993): 1–635.

Dufty, William. *Sugar Blues*. New York: Warner Books, 1976.

Guyton, Arthur C. *Textbook of Medical Physiology*. 7th ed. Philadelphia: W.B. Saunders, 1986.

Heaton, K. W., S. N. Mareus, P. M. Emmett, and C. H. Bolton. "Particle Size of Wheat, Maize and Oat Test Meals: Effects on Plasma, Glucose and Insulin Responses and on the Rate of Starch Digestion in Vitro." *American Journal of Clinical Nutrition* 47 (1988): 675–682.

Holmes, F. L. *Lavoisier and Chemistry of Life*. Madison: University of Wisconsin Press, 1985.

Jenkins D.J.A., et. al. "Glycemic Index of Foods: A Physiological Basis for Carbohydrate Exchange." *American Journal of Clinical Nutrition* 34 (1981): 362–66.

Jenkins D.J.A., et. al. "Low Glycemic Index Diet in Hyperlipidemia: Use of Traditional Starchy Foods." *American Journal of Clinical Nutrition* 46 (1987): 66–71.

Kahn, C. R., and G. C. Weir. *Joslin's Diabetes Mellitus*. 13th ed. Philadelphia: Lea and Febiger, 1994.

Knowler, W. C., D. J. Pettitt, M. F. Saad, and P. H. Bennett. "Diabetes Mellitus in the Pima Indians: Incidence, Risk Factors and Pathogenesis." *Diabetes and Metabolism Review* 6 (1990): 1–27.

Liebel, R. L., Rosenbaum, and J. Hirsch. "Changes in Energy Expenditure Resulting from Altered Body Weight." *New England Journal of Medicine* 332 (1995): 621.

Marmot, M., and E. Brunner. "Alcohol and Cardiovascular Disease: The Status of the U-Shaped Curve (Modified)." *British Medical Journal* 303 (1991): 565–568, figure 3.

Miller, Jennie B., Kaye Foster-Powell, and Stephen Colagiuri. *The G.I. Factor.* Rydalmere, Australia: Hodder Headline Australia PTY, Ltd., 1996.

Montignac, Michel. *Dine Out & Lose Weight.* Paris: Artulen, 1991.

Montignac, Michel. *Le Method Montignac Special Femme.* Paris: Artulen, 1994.

O'Keefe Jr., J. J., C. J. Lavie Jr., and B. D. McCallister. "Insights into the Pathogenesis and Prevention of Coronary Artery Disease." *Mayo Clinic Proceedings* 70 (1995): 69–79.

Skrabanek, Peti. "FatHeads." *National Review* 43 (1995): 43–47.

Webb, P. "The Measurement of Energy Exchange in Man, an Analysis." *American Journal of Clinical Nutrition* 33(6) (1980): 1299–1310.

World Health Organization. WHO Technical Report Series. "Cardiovascular Disease Risk Factors: New Areas for Research." Geneva 1994: 841.

Willis, Thomas. *Pharmaceutica Rationalis.* 1647.

Wilson, J. D., and D. W. Foster. *Williams Textbook of Endocrinology.* 8th ed. Philadelphia: W.B. Saunders, 1992.

Wolever, T.M.S., et al. "Beneficial Effects of Low-Glycemic Index Diet in Overweight NIDDM Subjects." *Diabetes Care* 15 (1992): 562–564.

Index

H. Leighton Steward has a master of science degree from Southern Methodist University and became CEO of a Fortune 500 energy company. He also authored a booklet on the causes of land loss of the lower Mississippi River wetland system. Sixty thousand of these booklets are in circulation worldwide and are referred to by many educational and governmental institutions. He is on the board of Tulane University as well as on several corporate boards. His own success and the success of others on this way of eating motivated him to write SUGAR BUSTERS!

Morrison C. Bethea, M.D., is a graduate of Davidson College and Tulane University School of Medicine. He completed his postgraduate training in thoracic and cardiac surgery at Columbia Presbyterian Medical Center in New York. Currently he practices thoracic, cardiac, and vascular surgery in New Orleans. He is the medical consultant to Freeport-McMoRan, Inc., for its worldwide operations and sits on the board of Taylor Energy and Tenet's Memorial Medical Center in New Orleans. Dr. Bethea has authored many publications in the field of cardiovascular disease and is a diplomate of the American Board of Thoracic Surgery.

Samuel S. Andrews, M.D., is a graduate of Louisiana State University School of Medicine. He currently practices internal medicine with the Audubon Internal Medicine Group. Dr. Andrews has authored many publications and participated in several drug studies in the field of endocrinology. He is a fellow in the American

Colleges of Physicians and Endocrinology. He is a clinical associate professor of medicine at Louisiana State University and a member of the pancreatic transplant team.

Luis A. Balart, M.D., is a graduate of Louisiana State University School of Medicine. He completed training in gastroenterology at Ochsner Clinic in New Orleans and in hepatology at the University of Southern California in Los Angeles. Dr. Balart practices gastroenterology and hepatology at Tenet's Memorial Medical Center in New Orleans and is clinical associate professor of medicine at Louisiana State University in New Orleans. He is currently involved in several clinical trials in the treatment of chronic viral hepatitis and is medical director of the Louisiana State University Liver Transplant Program.